Expert Pole Dancing

For Fitness and Fun

By

Danni Peck

Expert Pole Dancing: For Fitness and Fun

Copyright © 2017

All rights reserved. This book or any portion thereof may not be reproduced or used in any manner whatsoever without the express written permission of the publisher except for the use of brief quotations in a book review.

ISBN-10: 1521206384

ISBN-13: 978-1521206386

Warning and Disclaimer

Every effort has been made to make this book as accurate as possible. However, no warranty or fitness is implied. The information provided is on an "as-is" basis. The author and the publisher shall have no liability or responsibility to any person or entity with respect to any loss or damages that arise from the information in this book.

Publisher contact

Skinny Bottle Publishing

books@skinnybottle.com

Introduction 1
Extreme grip Mounts 2
    Elbow Flag to Flag 2
    Chinese Flag 4
    Chinese Flag with Attitude Legs 6
    Flag Back Roll 8
    Flag to Hip Lock 10
    Arms Only Pole Climb 12
    Down splits Variant 14
    Twisted Monkey 16
    Pointer 18
    One Arm Embrace 20
    Arms Only climb Straddle 22
Expert Inverts 24
    Split Grip Chinese Rubber Aysha 24
    Straight Edge to Shoulder Mount 26
    Twisted Chinese Flag 28
    U-Bend 30
    La Roue 32
    Rubber Double elbow 34
    Allegra Box splits 36
    Banana split 38
    Bendy diva dive 40
    Death lay 42
Extreme Poses 45

  Chopsticks 46

  Rocket man 48

  Planche 50

  Iron X 52

  Extended Flexi Embrace 54

Extreme Doubles Actions to Master 56

  One armed inverted one leg hang 56

  One arm inverted straddle 58

  Circle 60

  Two-Partnered Handspring 62

  Death K 64

How to Build Flexibility 66

Tips to Help with Recording your Pole Moves 72

  Mirror, mirror 72

  Put it on Video 73

  Practice Makes Perfect 74

That's It! 75

Introduction

You've mastered the beginner work, gotten the hang of intermediate, were able to rock the advanced moves, now it's time for the expert pole training moves to try.

This book gives you a comprehensive array of amazing pole moves to master. With each of these, they do take a bit of time to learn and master, and with every single trick, you'll be able to truly get all of the great results from this as you go along.

Pole dancing is an art, an art that you should work to master. It does take time, and you might get mad at yourself, but as you continue working on this, and with these expert moves at your disposal, you'll be able to really get the most out of your ability to learn this, and because of that, you'll feel way better as well.

I took a lot of time to learn each of these moves, and they are definitely not for the ones who haven't done it before. They require a lot of strength and flexibility, which we'll go over in a later chapter as well. It's time to learn into this wide array of pole moves, and see what you can accomplish.

Extreme grip Mounts

Now, with pole dancing, mounting your body and holding it there can be quite hard. However, there are some pretty amazing and interesting tricks to try out, epically if you're looking for something way more challenging. These tricks require a strong amount of arm strength, but they are certainly worth it if you're looking to really take your pole dancing to a new height. With each move, you can spend time learning it, and once you master it, you can move onto the next one.

Elbow Flag to Flag

Now this one is one of the tricks that looks easy, but it's all arm strength and gripping. To begin, have your outer arm against the pole at a higher level, holding it there around the elbow area. You want to nestle this against the crook of the elbow. Take your other hand, and put it in the position you would for a wide grip. You then kick off, hold it there, and then, when you're comfortable, immediately take your top hand and slide the hand over to a standard wide grip. Maintain that hold. Now this one might be easier to learn first if you master both the elbow flag and the standard flag, then combining them. Typically, the elbow flag is a bit easier to learn initially.

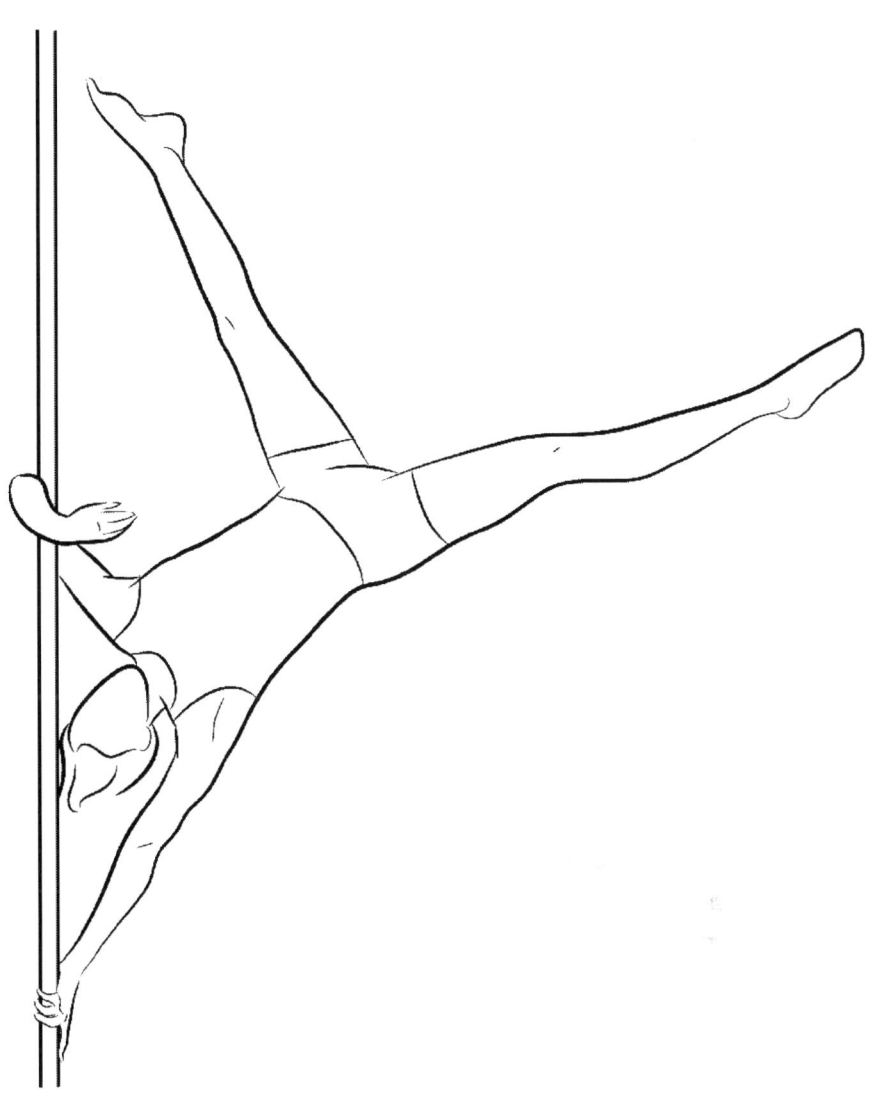

Chinese Flag

This is a move that is a great one to learn initially when you're trying to do these variants. To begin, you should have your arms in the wide grip once more. Ideally, your pole should be in the static placement, not moving about. from there, kick your legs up, bring them as high as you can, almost inverting the body. You can rely on the pole for beginning practice, but try to have it so it's just far enough away that it's not touching the pole. From there, you can bring the legs outward and hold it there. This is a complex move, and if you don't have the arm and ab strength, it's encouraged to start working on that as well.

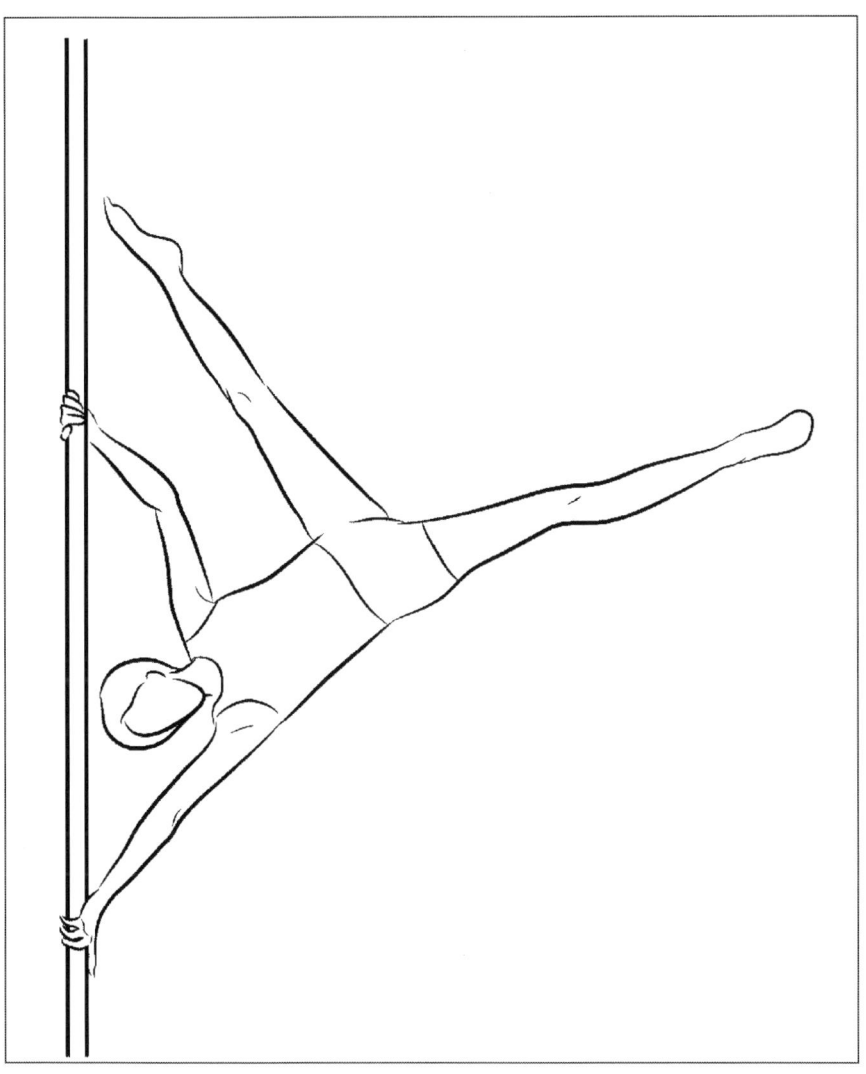

Chinese Flag with Attitude Legs

The Chinese flag is one of the harder moves to try, but adding the attitude legs can certainly make it look even more amazing. To begin, you take your dominant hand and put it on top, and then the other hand on the bottom. You should use a wide grip for this. From there, you should kick your legs off, using your core to help you balance, and from there, once you have that, bring your legs together, with one bent and the other straightened. This takes a lot of work to get used to and requires not only arm, but also ab strength.

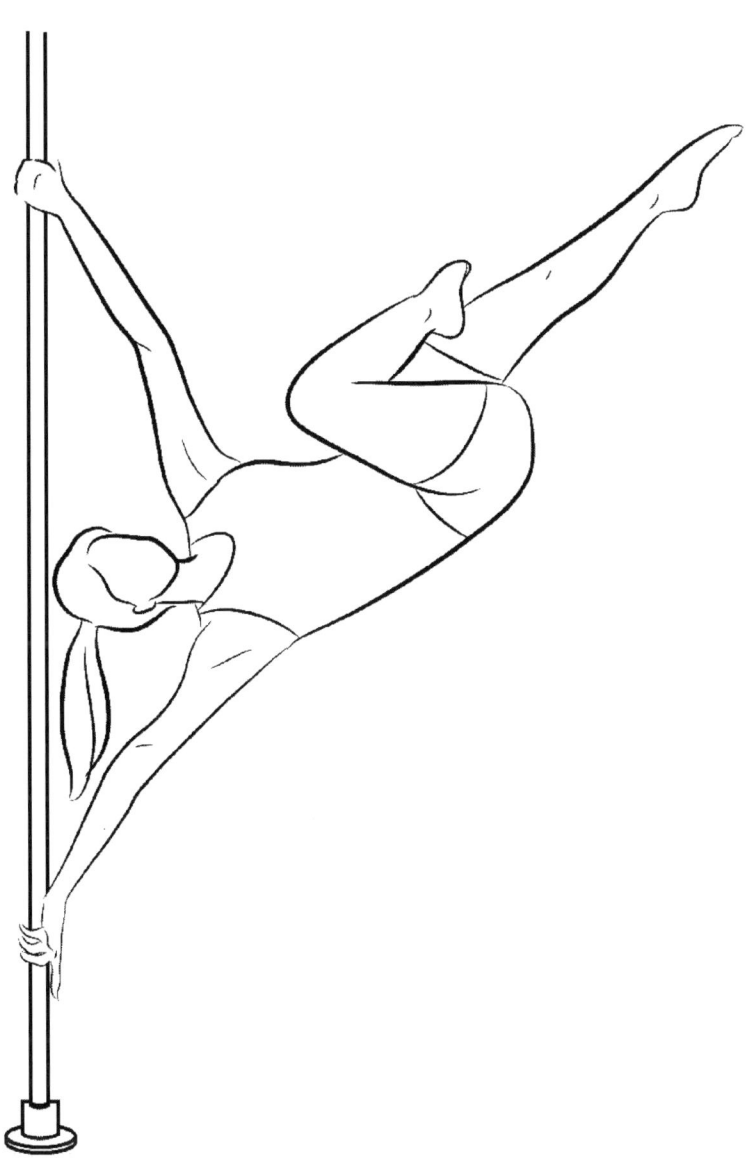

Flag Back Roll

This is another flag variant. To do this, you want to get into the flag position. however, this time, you will want to move your body around. Once you get up there, you bring your legs behind you and slide them behind, twisting your hands in the process so you don't hurt yourself. For some, they can learn this move immediately on a spinning pole, but for others, it might be best to begin in a static pole so you don't und up dizzying yourself. This one takes a bit longer to learn, simply because you are moving, but it is an incredibly fun move to try out.

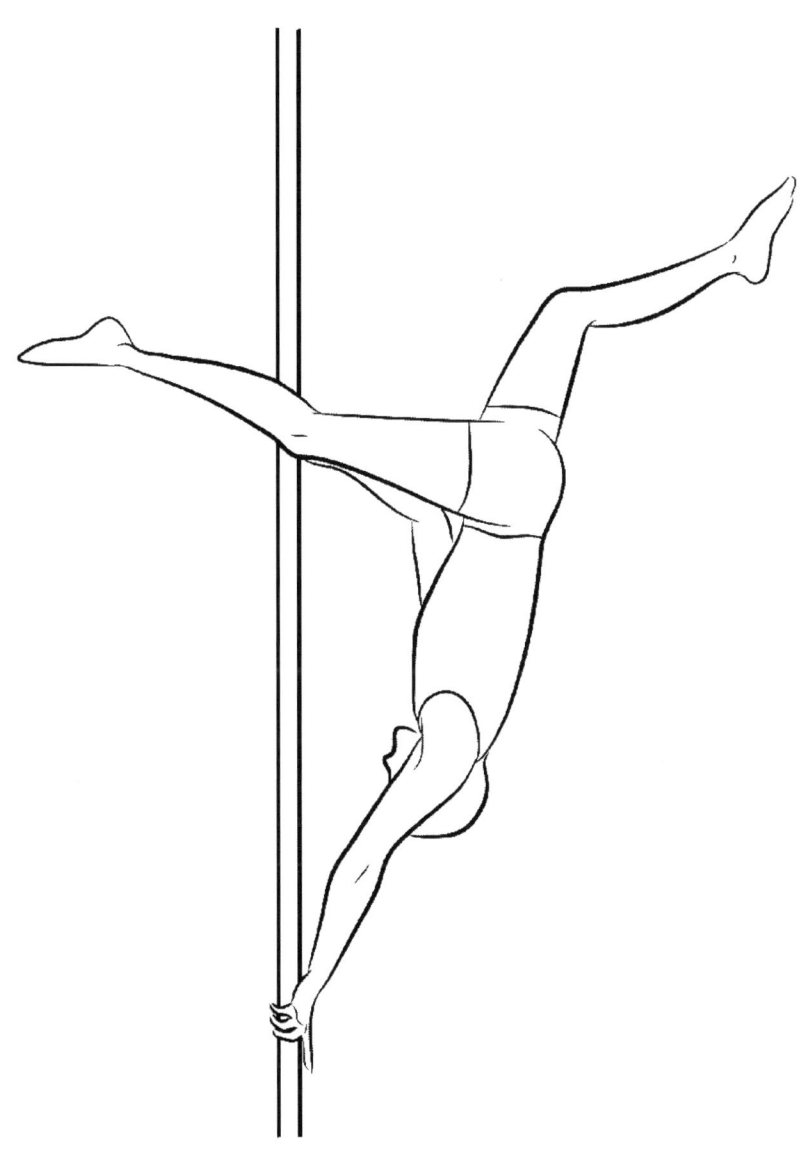

Flag to Hip Lock

This is another flag variant, but it changes into something else. To begin, you want to start in a flag position. You should get up into that. however, instead of bringing your legs down, you wrap them over, hugging the pole and then locking your hips onto there. You should then bring your legs close, sliding down the pole. This is another extremely hard move, and it should only be attempted once you are able to achieve the other moves listed before this.

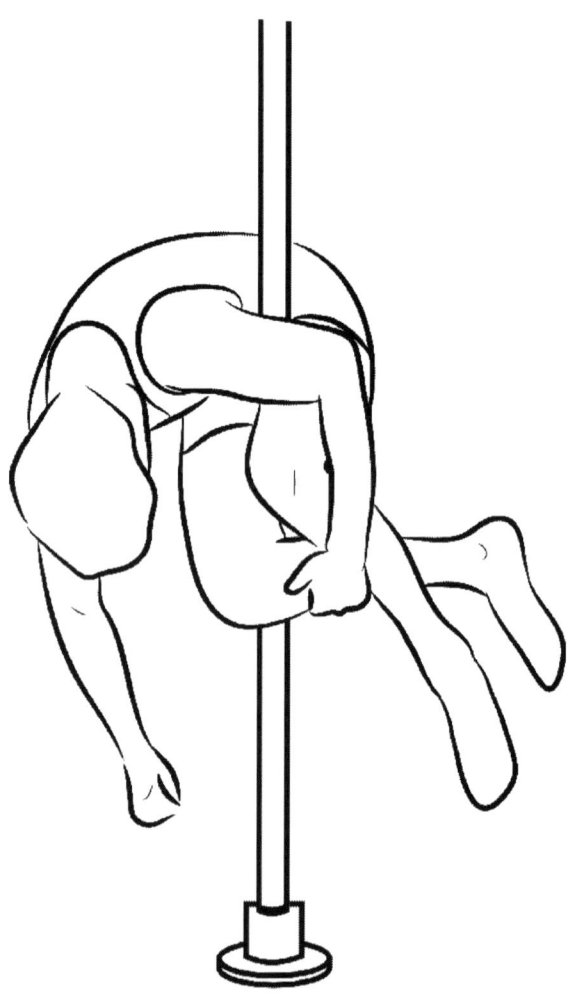

Arms Only Pole Climb

To do this, you want to completely rely on arm strength. To start, you want to put each leg against the pole and your hands in a basic grip. From there, wrap them around the pole, but try not to touch it completely. You then take your arms and start to climb. This is one of those moves that isn't necessarily hard because of the technique, but it requires a significant amount of arm strength. This is a great arm building exercise if you're looking for something that will really help.

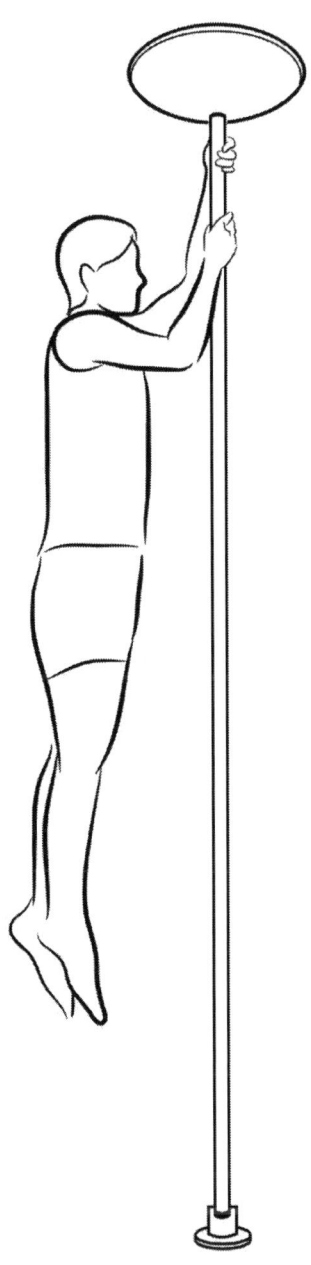

Down splits Variant

This is a variant of down splits. Some might like this, but it requires much more arm and ab strengthen than your typical down splits. To begin, you want to start in a basic inversion. Once you do that, you should wrap a leg around, preferably the left, and then take the right and have it completely straighten out against the pole. Unwrap the bent leg, and from there, slowly push your arms down. Once you're at the same level as your arms, you should then proceed to extend your leg out, holding it there. This is a much harder version of a typical down split, but this is something that certainly does look great, and the crispness of it does make it look really amazing as well.

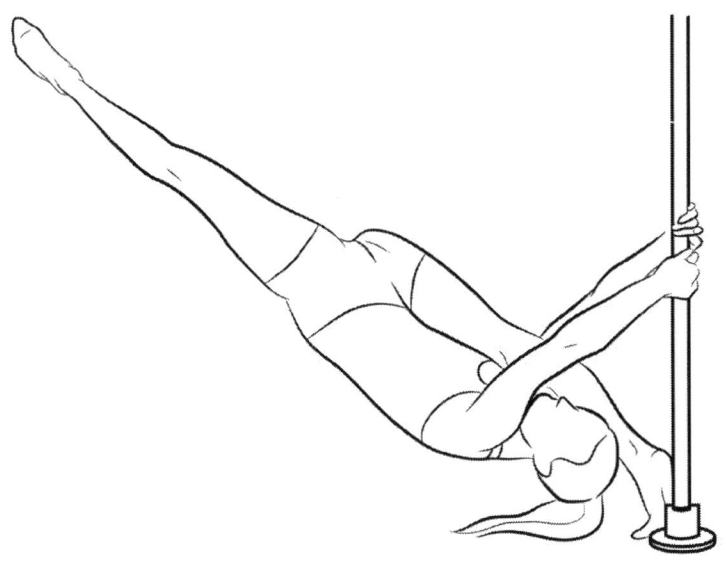

Twisted Monkey

This is very similar to the elbow flag in a sense. To begin, you should have your left arm against the pole at the elbow level, and the other in a wide grip. You should kick your legs up, holding it there, and from there, you should proceed to take your legs and put them almost in a stag position. Take your elbow, and start to put your hand against the base of your ankle, and the other on your ankle in the front. You should have it set so that your knee is bracing your body against the pole along with your inner right arm. This is a hard move to learn, but when you do learn the basic flag and master it, this makes it a whole lot easier for many.

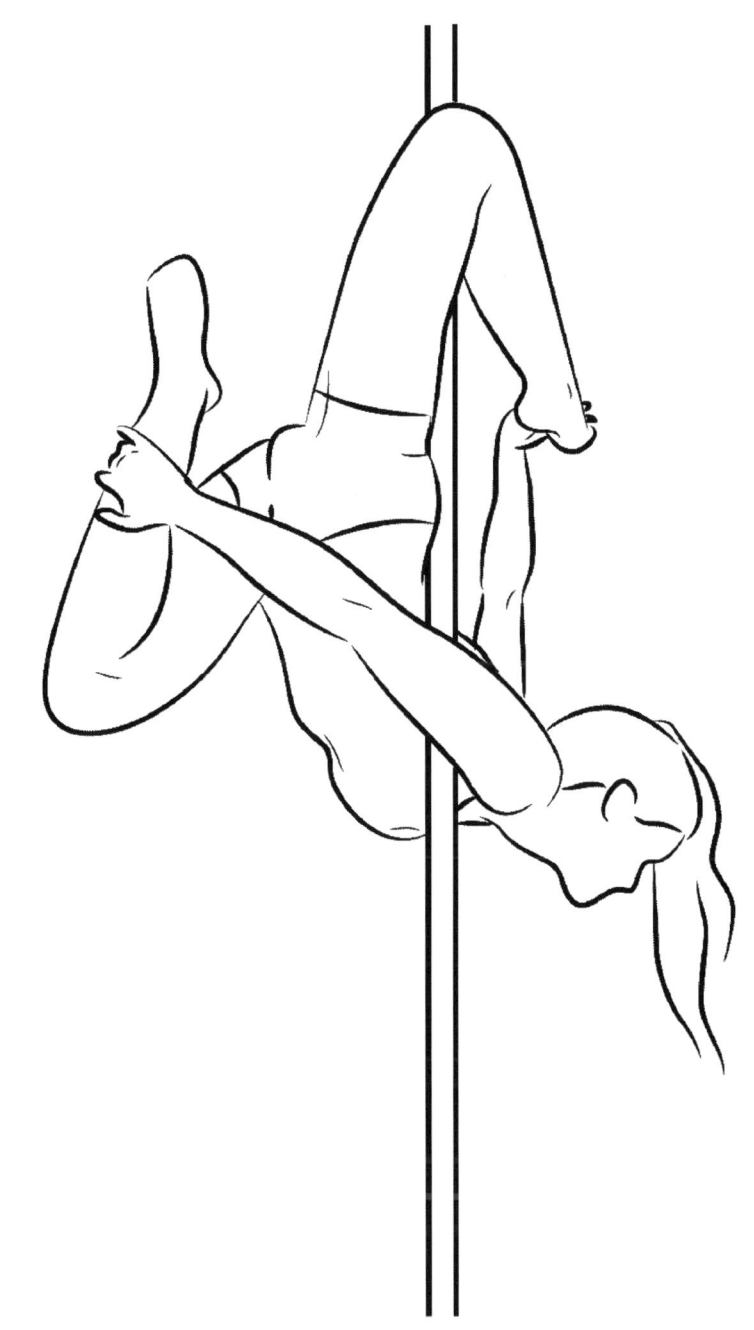

Pointer

This is similar to many of the flag variants, but the biggest difference is how you're gripping. Instead of the typical wide grip, you're using a reverse grip to hold yourself up, with your right hand facing outward and your wrist twisted inward, with your left arm against the bottom. You should then kick up, and from there, hold the position. it might take a minute for you to maintain this, but you should then start to press your legs forward, holding them there in a pointed position. This is a move that will take a bit of time to learn, especially since the gripping is much different from your typical move. However, this is a lot of fun, and it can be quite the move to learn if you're looking for a challenge.

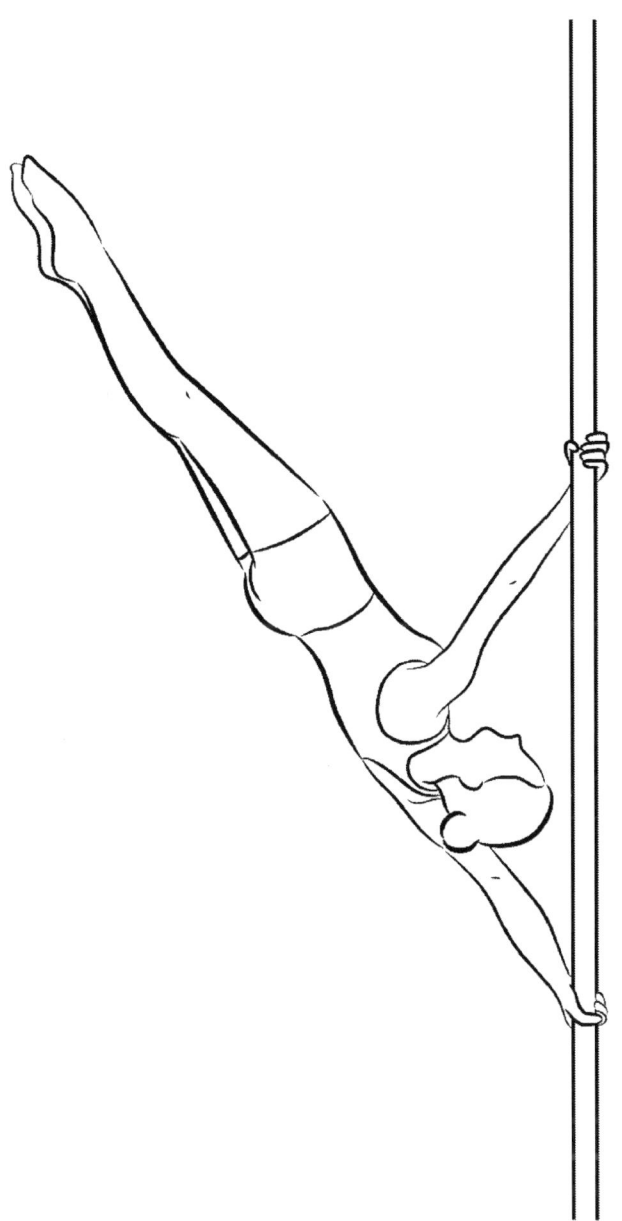

One Arm Embrace

This is a variant of another move discussed in the advanced pole tricks book. To begin, you should climb the pole, with your right arm using the elbow area and your left arm on tops. Once you have climbed up, take your legs and put them with the feet touching one another at the bottoms. It should make almost a triangular position. Then, slowly take your other arm off. You want to be off of the pole, letting your elbow hold all of the weight and gripping it. This is a great way to improve your strength, especially if you struggle with holding your body up at the elbow level. If you're going to learn the flag, you should try this first.

Another fun thing you can do is that you can take your other hand, and climb up, using your elbow as support. You can go higher, remove it, and continue this for a great climbing move that definitely tests your grips.

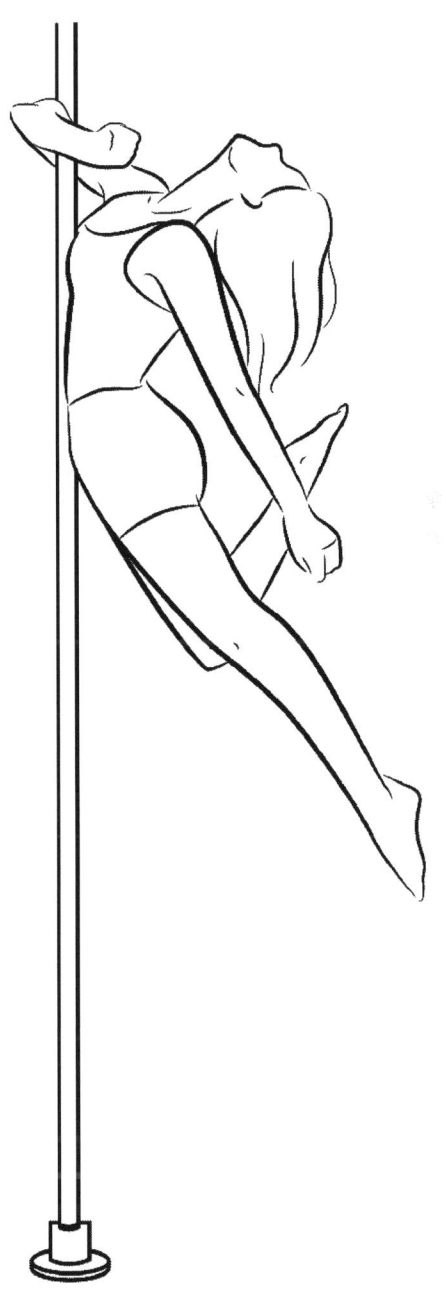

Arms Only climb Straddle

This is another great climb to learn, especially if you're wanting to learn how to climb with only your hands to assist you. however, instead of having your legs against the pole, they will be straddled out to the side, the opposite side of your hands. To begin, have your hands in a basic grip, then kick off your legs and have them at the side. You can then straddle them from side to side if you want as you begin to climb. This is incredibly difficult, but it's a climbing move that will certainly test your arm strength if you're looking for one that does. If you're looking to improve your grips as well, this is perfect for you too.

With all of these grips and climbs, it's encouraged to learn them all static first. Often, we end up learning one way or another, but the thing is, when you're trying to learn how to do a flag, you need to have a good footing to begin with. Often when you're spinning and learning this, it can make it quite hard for you to really get anywhere with this. That's why, it's encouraged that you learn this on static, and once you feel ready, do this on a spinning pole. Also, don't try to learn all of these at once. The best way to go is to start with the flag variants, and from there, go to other movements that you can use. It will certainly help you, and it'll make it a lot easier for you to understand these moves that much more.

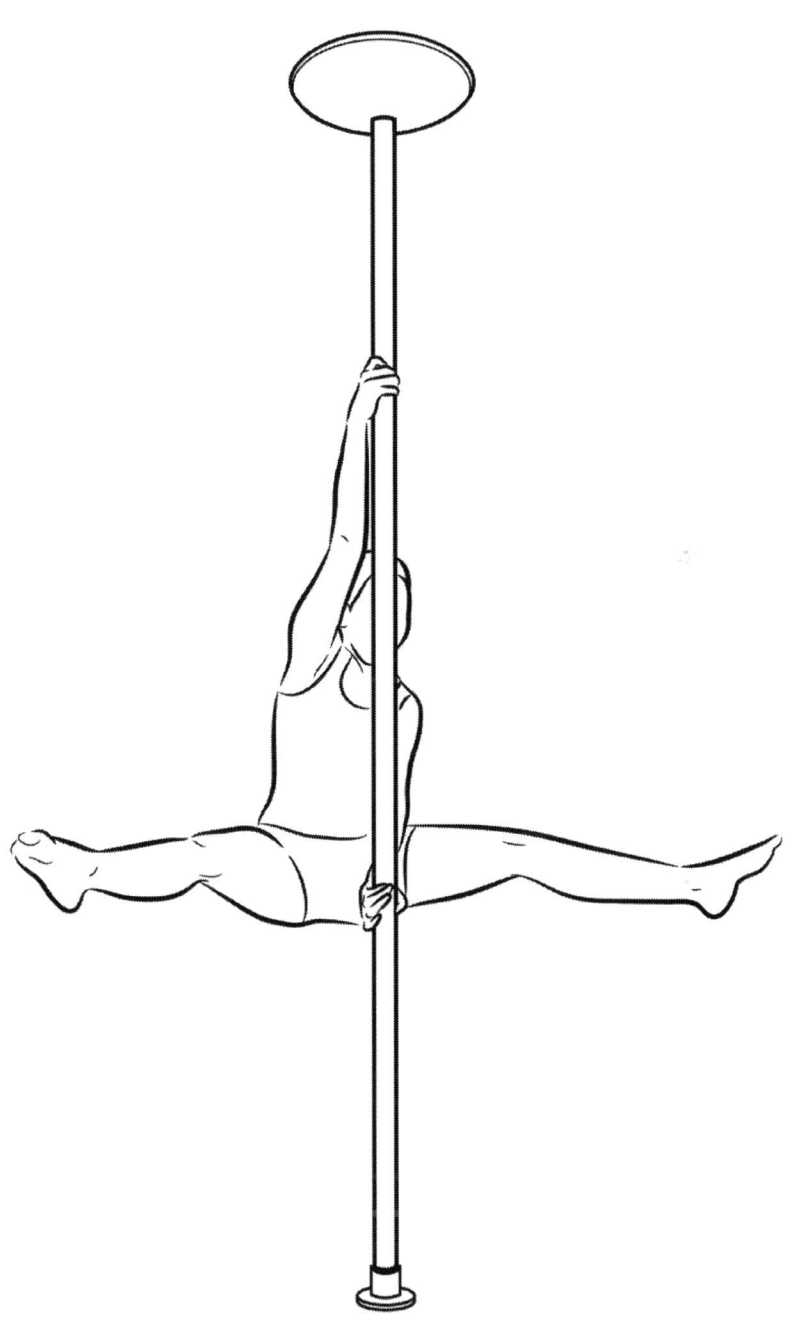

Expert Inverts

Inverts are even more fun, and way more challenging at the expert level. They require much more arm and ab strength than before, but it also requires some bravery too. This chapter will go over some of the expert inverts to try out, and what you need to do in order to master every single one of them in a simple, yet efficient manner.

Split Grip Chinese Rubber Aysha

This is a move that often requires you to not only know how to invert correctly but also, it's good to learn how to do a flag first since this does base itself off a flag. To begin, you want to go into a basic invert. From there, put your hands down into a split grip position. You should then take your legs and extend them outward, holding them together and bending them at the knee. This is where the ab strength comes in since you'll be balancing yourself up on the pole each time you do so. From there, in order to get down, you can either, let go and get back onto your feet if you're low, or take your legs, wrap them around, bring your hands together into a basic grip, and then slide down the pole. This does take a bit of practice and some getting used to, and you'll be able to learn this in no time if you have mastered the flag.

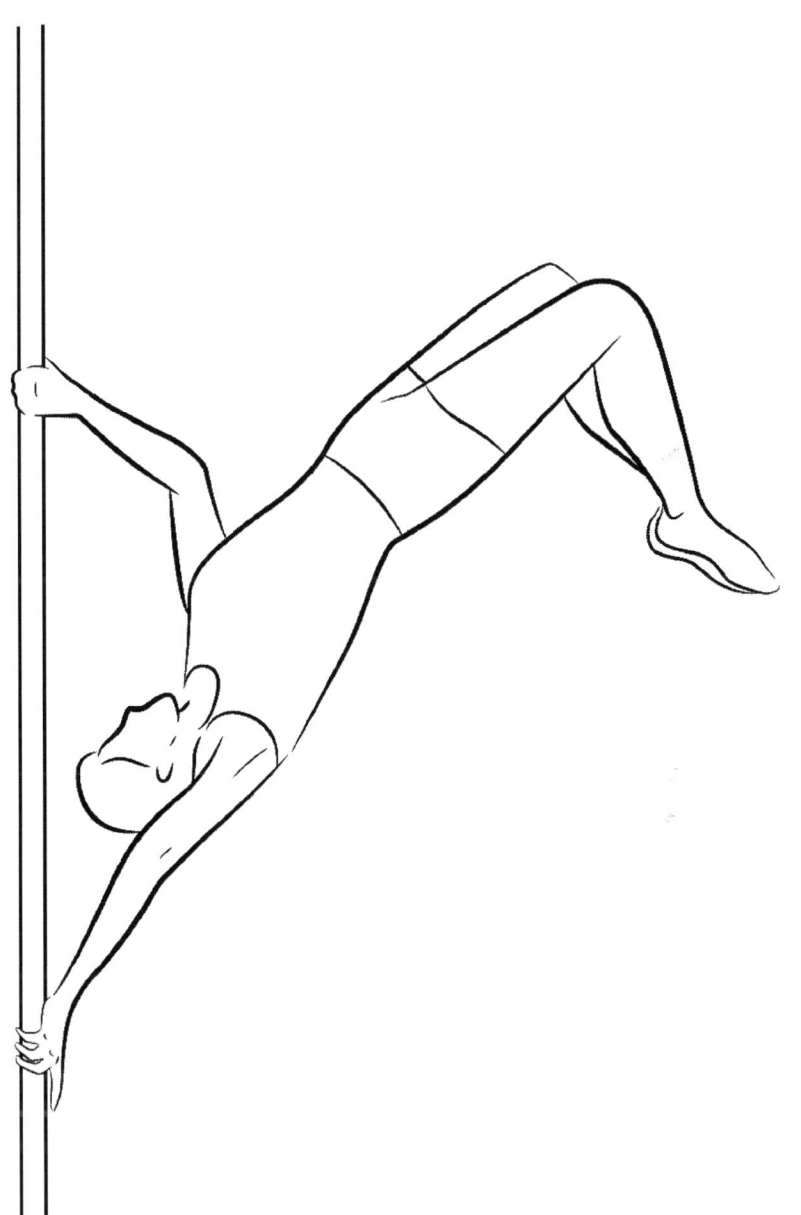

Straight Edge to Shoulder Mount

These are always really fun to do. To begin, you should get yourself into a basic invert, and from there, you want to straighten your body as straight as you can get. However, this is where it gets harder. Now, the biggest precaution about this is to try to get yourself high enough that you won't bang your head on the ground or on the little stage surrounding the pole. You want to take your legs, and from there, change your hand grip to a cup grip, pulling your legs off and pulling it down into a shoulder mount grip. You'll be very low to the ground, which is fine, that's how it works. This can be quite shocking initially since you might think you'll fall, but if you have your grips correct and have mastered the shoulder mount, you'll be fine.

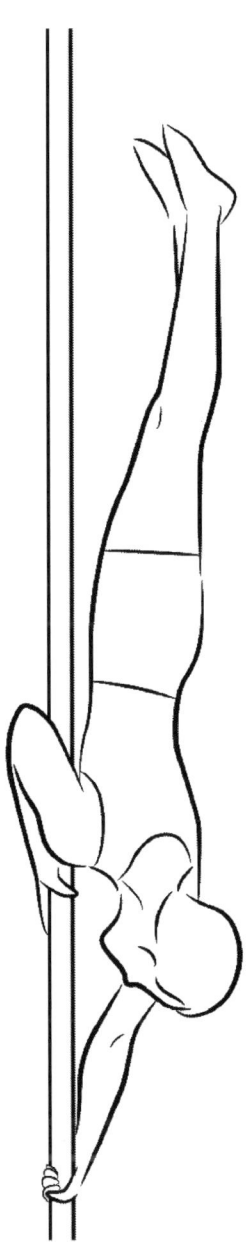

Twisted Chinese Flag

This is another variant of the Chinese flag. To begin, you want to get yourself into the Chinese flag position. from there, you want to simply take your legs, straighten them out, and cross them opposite of the direction your body is going, holding it there as you do so. This might feel weird, but compared to other variants, this is actually one of the easier ones. Once you are finished, you can simply move your body down by bringing your legs back to the other side that your hands are on, and laying them on the ground.

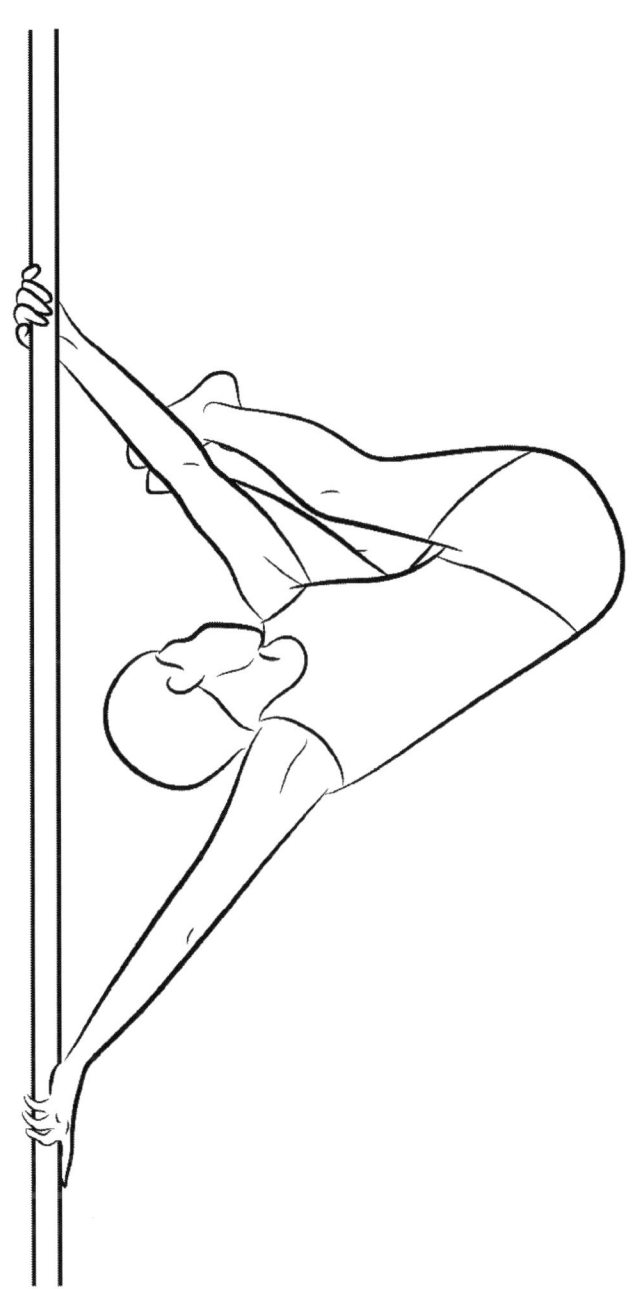

U-Bend

this move is a very complicated and kind of weird-looking move when you first look at it. To begin, you want to be in a standard grip, having your left leg against the bottom, and from there, taking your leg and extending it as far up the pole as you can go, holding it there. Now, here is where the fun begins. You want to take that upper leg, and wrap it opposite of the side your left leg is on. Change your hands from a basic grip to almost a cup grip. From there, you should climb the legs down in order to get them to the same level. Your torso will be facing outward. At this point, you should then take one of your hands off, holding it there in a pose. To get back off the pole, you can simply take your legs and split them outward, or just climb down the pole at this point.

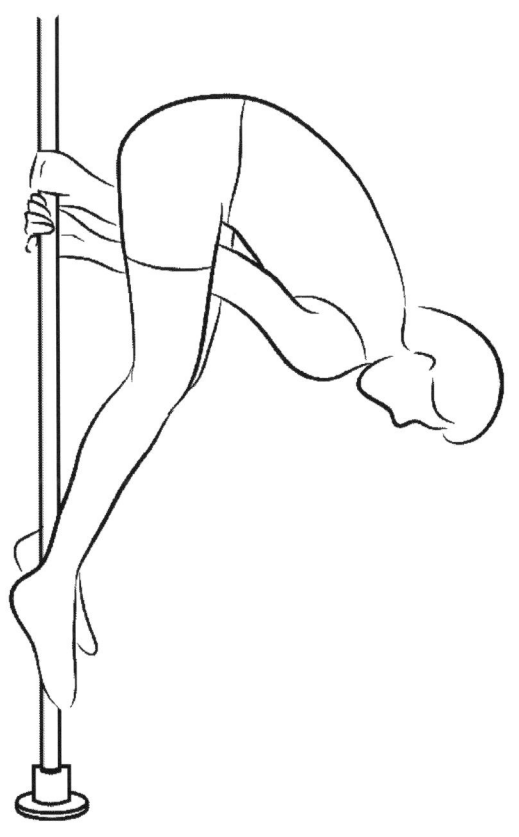

La Roue

This move is a fun little invert to try, and it is very similar to the u-bend. To begin, you want to put yourself in that same position, so do so. From there though, instead of just leaving your leg out, you want to extend it, hold it there, and then wrap it over your body to the other side. This is quite a complicated move, so keep that in mind when you are doing it. ideally, it's best to master the u-bend first before you try this one since it is a more complex version of it.

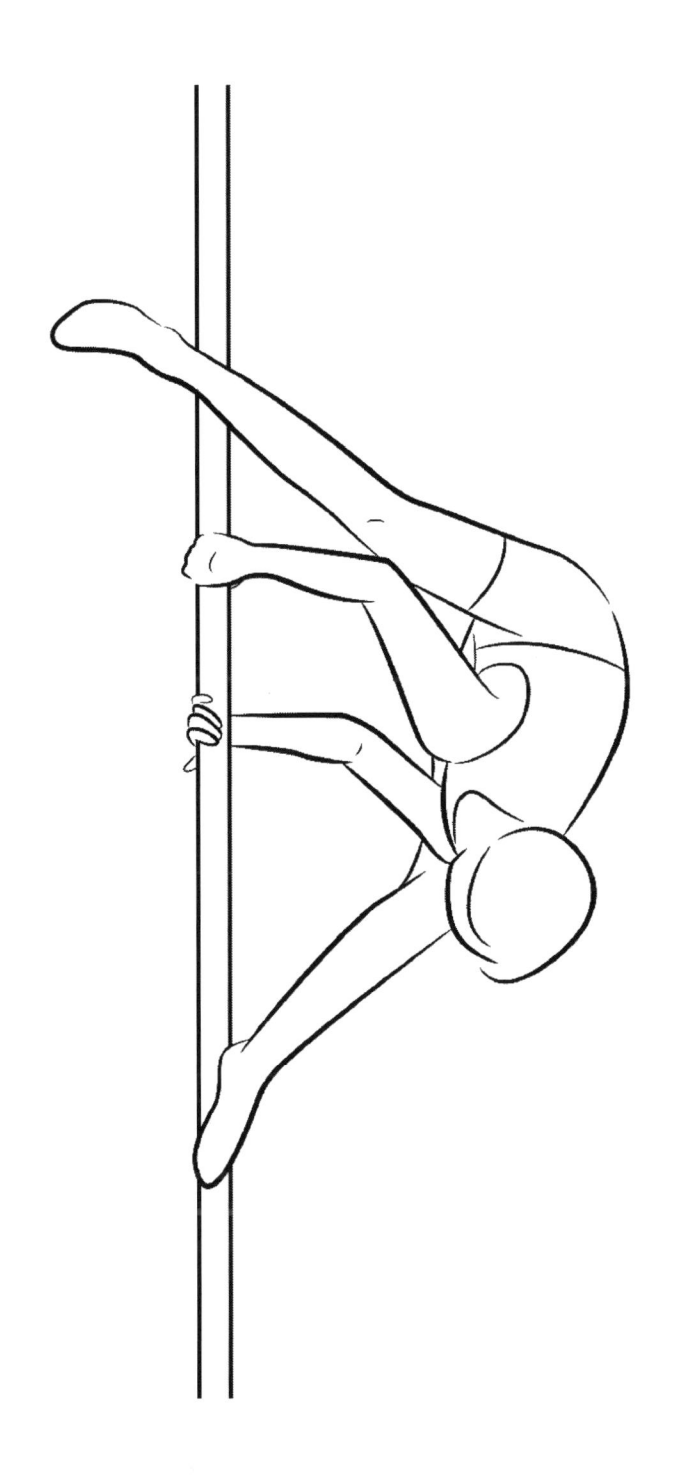

Rubber Double elbow

this move is a pretty, but very hard elbow grip move. To begin, you want to climb the pole, and then do a basic layback. However, at this point, you want to take your elbow, grip it behind the pole, and take your other hand and put it about a foot down. Then, you should take your legs, and slowly bend them, getting them as close to your backside and back as much as you can. From there, you can maintain the hold, or even take your legs and pull them forward, helping you to get off the pole.

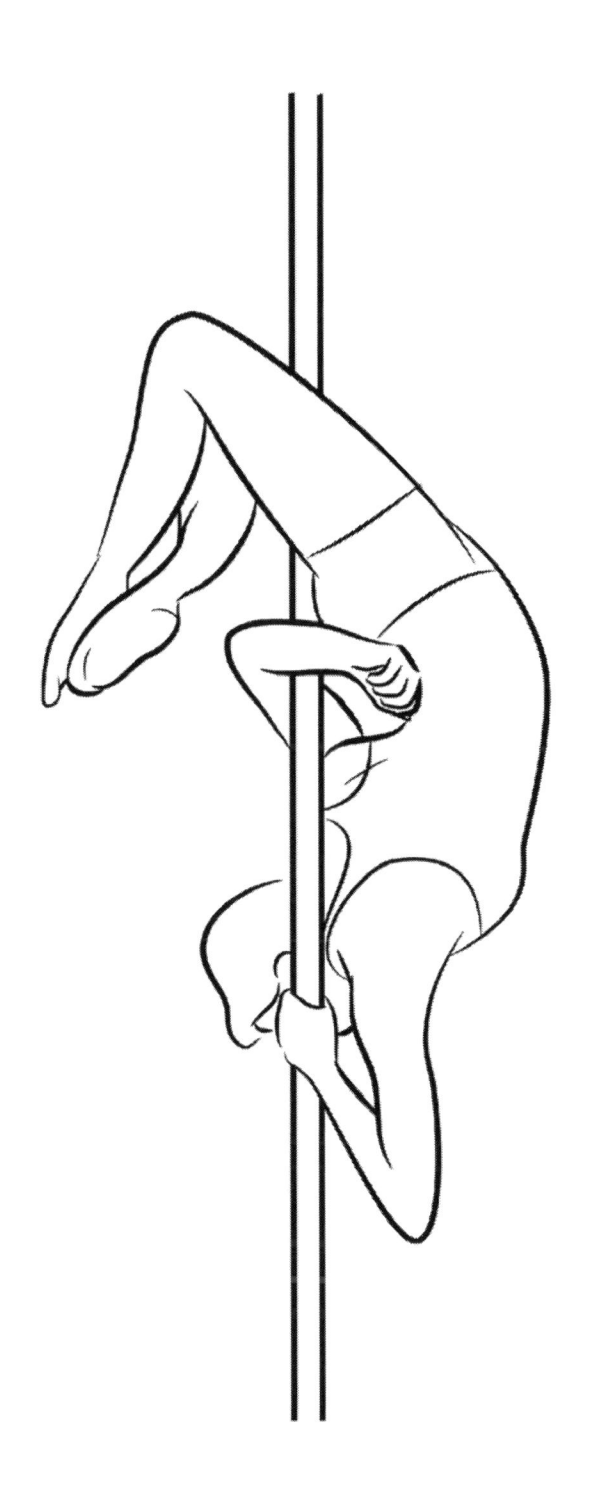

Allegra Box splits

If you are good at box splits and love to do allegras, then this variant is perfect for you. To begin, you want to be in a wide grip and then invert around the pole. Take your right leg, bend it over the pole, and then take your left leg and push it downwards. From there, you want to straighten it, take your torso, and bring it forward. From there, you want to take your top leg, and straighten it as far as you can possibly go, ideally to the point of a split. From there, you can hold it and then get down. Now, this move isn't simple, it's one that requires great flexibility, so it's encouraged that you master your own personal flexibility first before attempting this sort of move.

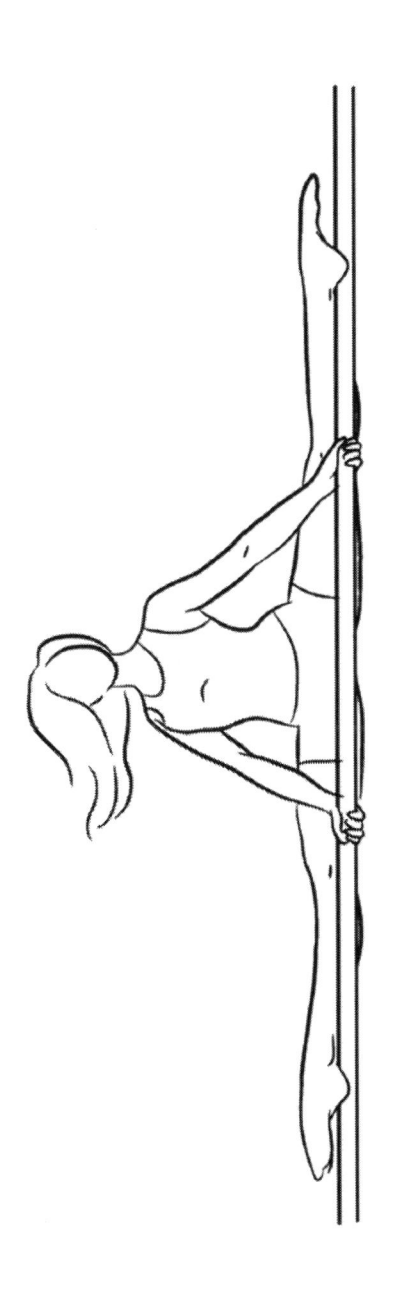

Banana split

This is a pole move that is similar in a sense to the splits talking about before. However, you're not going to go into an Allegra. To begin, you want to climb up and get into the basic invert. From there, take your left leg and put it around the pole at the knee area. Take your bottom leg, which should be your right, and from there, extend it out below you. move your body so that you're in a basic grip against the pole, and from there, slowly take your left leg and push it as outward as you can. If you have been working on your flexibility, this should be relatively easy for you to do, since you're able to extend it as far as possible. Your legs should be on different sides, so it's a bit simpler than the box splits.

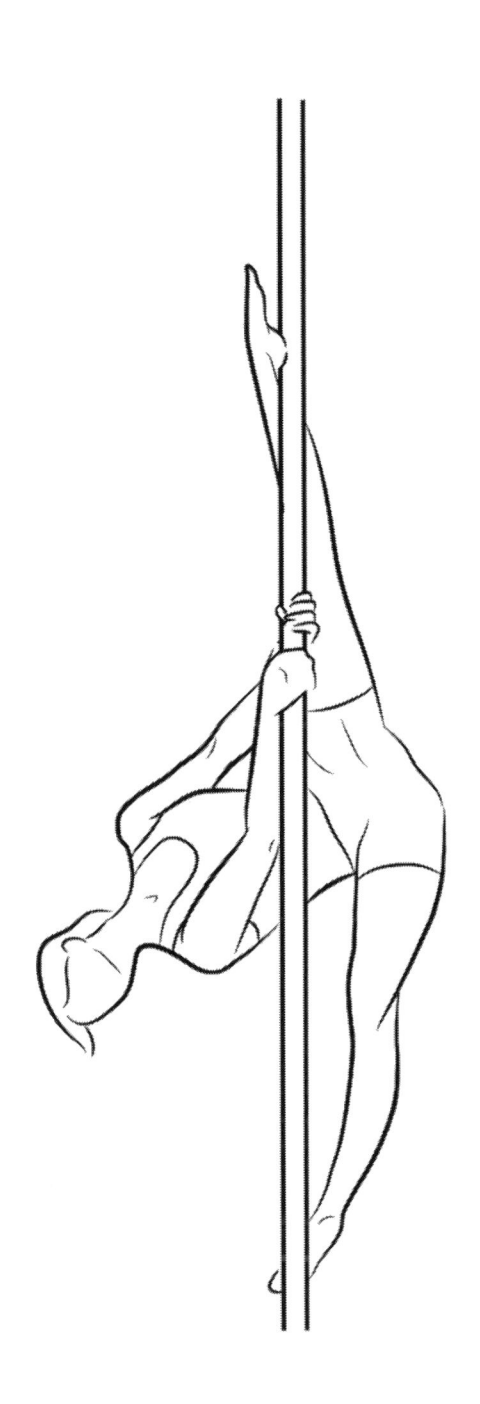

Bendy diva dive

This is a fun and bendy little trick you can try. To begin, you want to do a basic climb up the pole, and from there, begin to do a lay back. From there, you want to bring your body against the pole, with your left leg kept straight and gripping at the ankle and the upper thigh. From there, you want to take your other leg, bend it, and hold it there, extending your body. You can use both hands to grip this, or you can take one hand and put it over the other. This is a fun and simple bending invert move, and it's a good one to try if you're still trying to learn the expert pole moves.

41

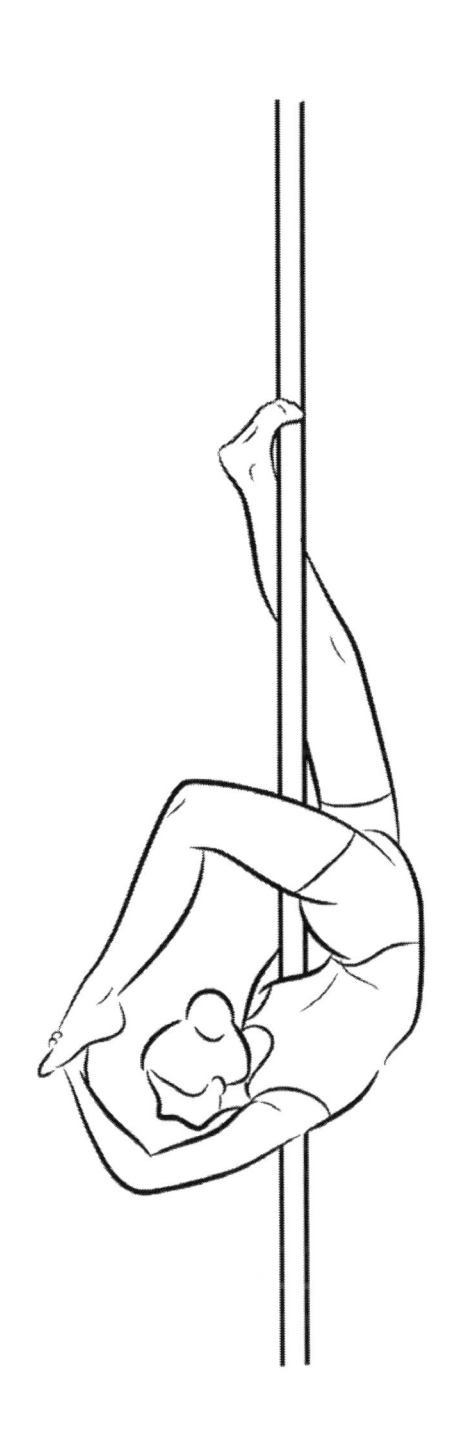

Death lay

The death lay is the final invert that we'll go over, and this one requires a bit of courage to do, not just skill. The reason for this is because you will be holding yourself against the pole with your torso to the ground. Some pole dancers actually like to drop from this, which is where the death drop comes from. I suggest not doing a death drop until you have full control of your drops, and you have mastered the death lay.

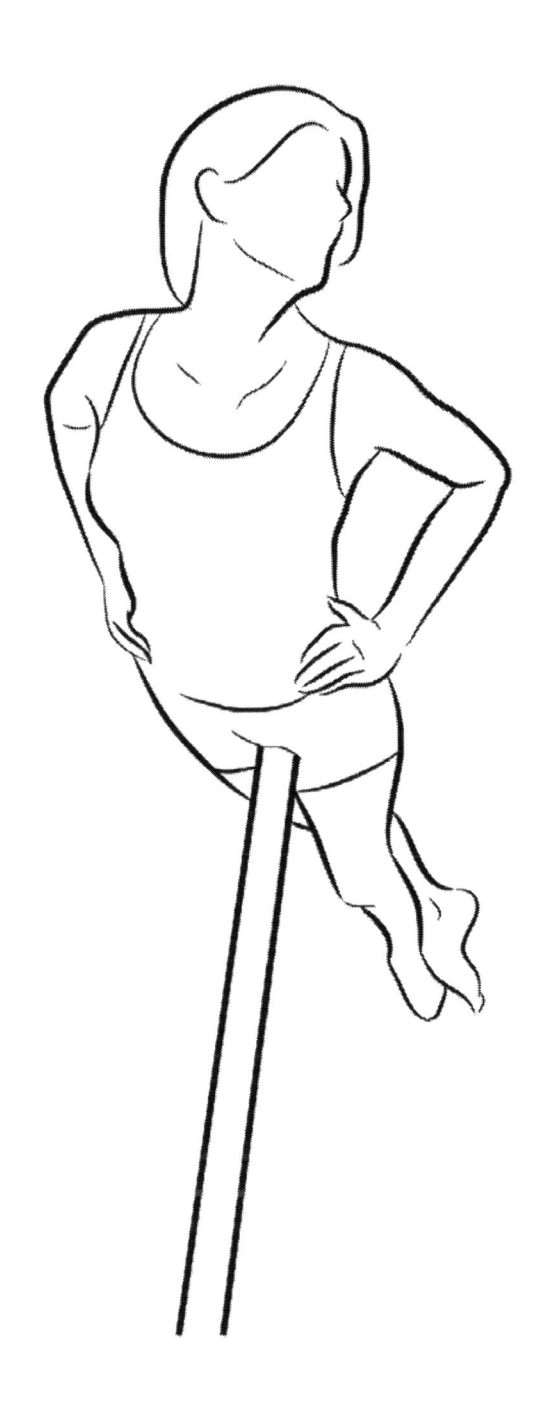

To begin, you can climb up the pole, and then take your legs and push it up into an invert. You can then climb your legs up, and from there, have your legs fall back a little bit so that they're extended outward. Get your legs climbed up to the same level, and from there, slowly take your arms off of the pole, holding it there as you use your thighs to grip it there. If you can't take both hands off of there immediately, do one at a time, for it will be much easier. If you want to learn the death drop, you can slowly take your thighs and pull them off, clenching them together before you hit the ground. However, it's a very dangerous move and shouldn't be attempted unless you either have mastered this, or have someone that is nearby to help in case if you do end up overestimating it.

These inverts are much harder than your average move, but they can be done. You can try each of these mastering them every single time. You may never know what you can do until you try these, so have a shot at them, for they are a lot of fun.

Extreme Poses

Posing on the pole is something that many people want to get better at, but it does take a bit of time and effort to master. This chapter will go over some great poses to master in order to take your pole work to the next level.

Chopsticks

The chopsticks is a fun and complicated pole move. To begin, you want to climb up onto the pole, and from there, wrap your arm around the front holding the pole with your armpit. From there, take your bottom hand and hold it there in a basic grip. For your legs, take your right one and extend it out, and then do the same with your left. Essentially, you almost want to get into the splits, but not completely. From there, you can hold it, making it easier for you to maintain. When finished, bring your legs together, and slide down the pole.

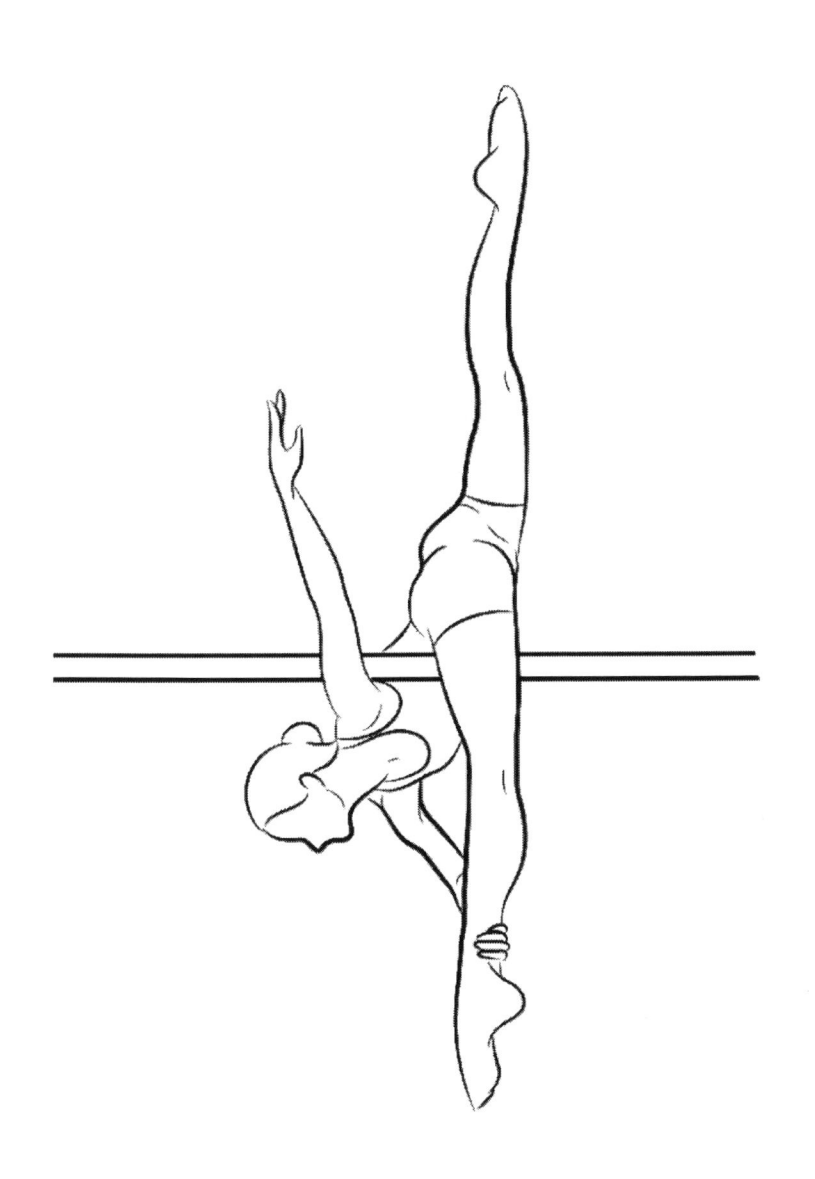

Rocket man

This is a fun pole dancing pose to try out. Essentially, what you want to do is climb up the pole, take your inner hand, and wrap it around. You should have it right against the pole in a straight manner, in line with your body. From there, take your legs and hold them back, maintaining your hold against the pole. From there, bring your other arm to the side as well. This isn't super complicated compared to the other moves, but it is a nice pose to learn and add to your routine.

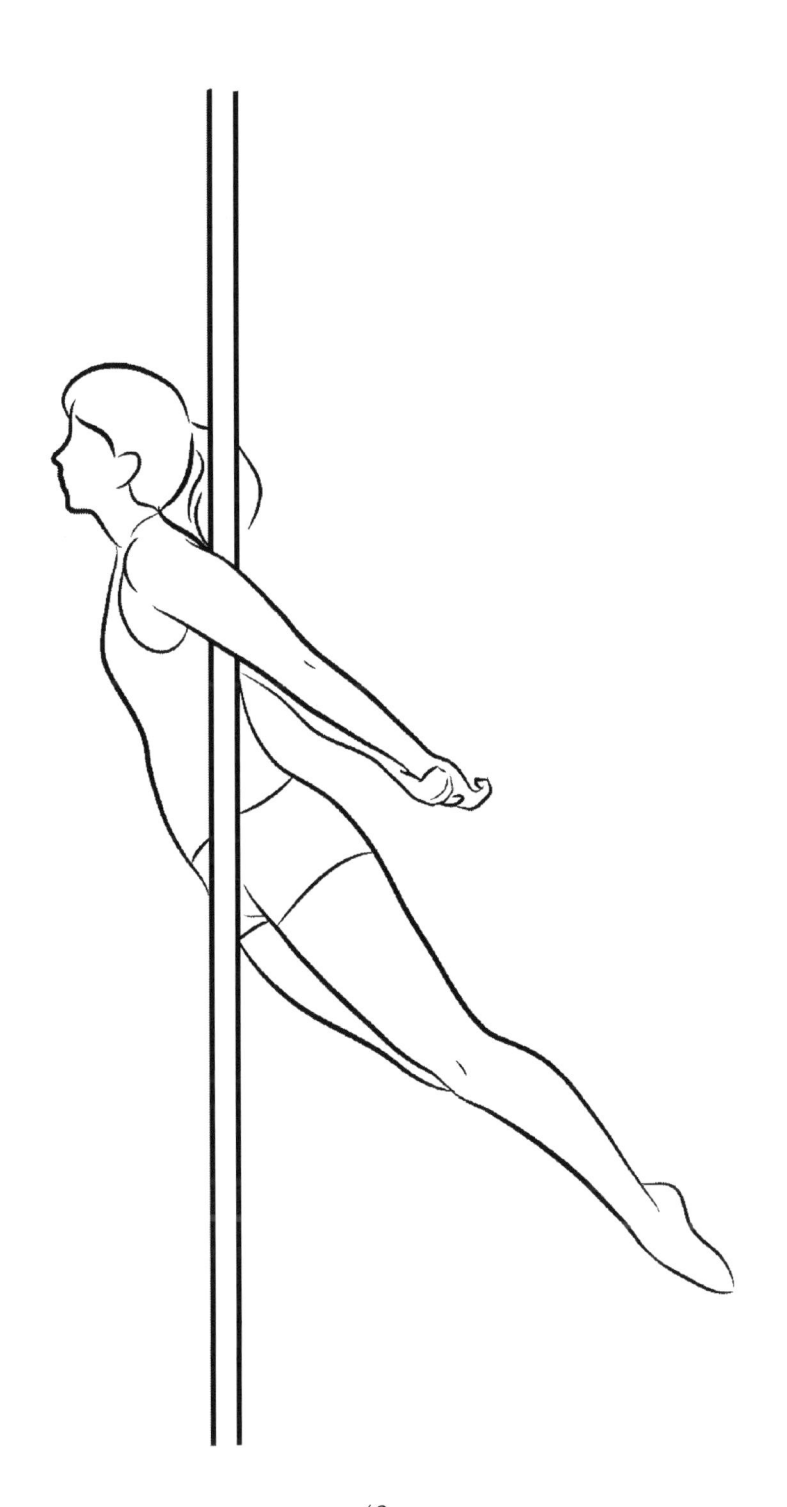

Planche

The planche is a very hard inverted move. To begin. You want to climb up the pole, and then, get as far to the top as you can. You actually want to be at the very top of your pole. If you're using a stage pole, get to where the end of it is. From there, you want to hold the pole in a basic grip, have half of your torso over it, and then push your legs back, extending them either over your body or in line with your body. You should then proceed to hold it there.

Now, this move is very complicated, and it shouldn't be attempted unless you've worked at that level of the pole. Along with this, you have to be very careful with the body weight as well, since it might move a little bit. If you want to try it, do take some time to practice it, but don't jump all the way to the top right away, go from smaller levels up.

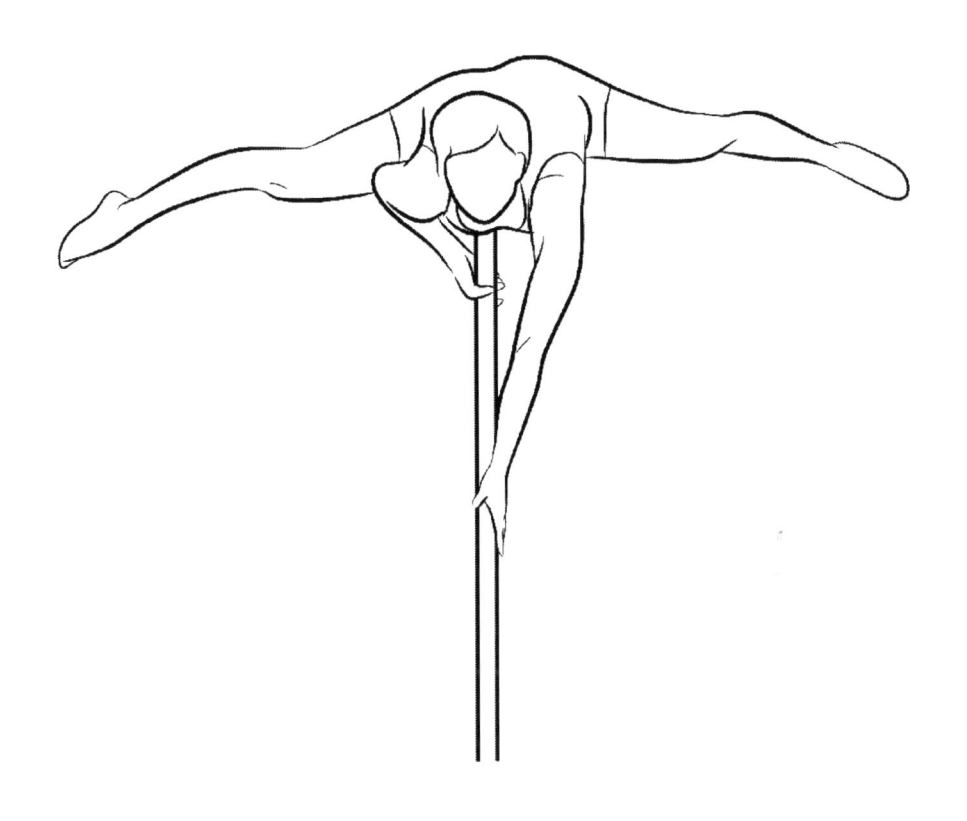

Iron X

The iron X is a great pole move to try, and for a pole move at an expert level, it's pretty simple. If you know how to do a flag, you're already well on your way to learning this. Essentially, you want to have an extended grip on the pole, and from there, you should kick your legs up, spreading them into an X position. from there, you want to maintain a hold on the pole there. This one is a great one if you're looking for a great pose that will add to your routine. If you want to, try the flags first, and from there, move onto this, for it will make it much easier for you when you do.

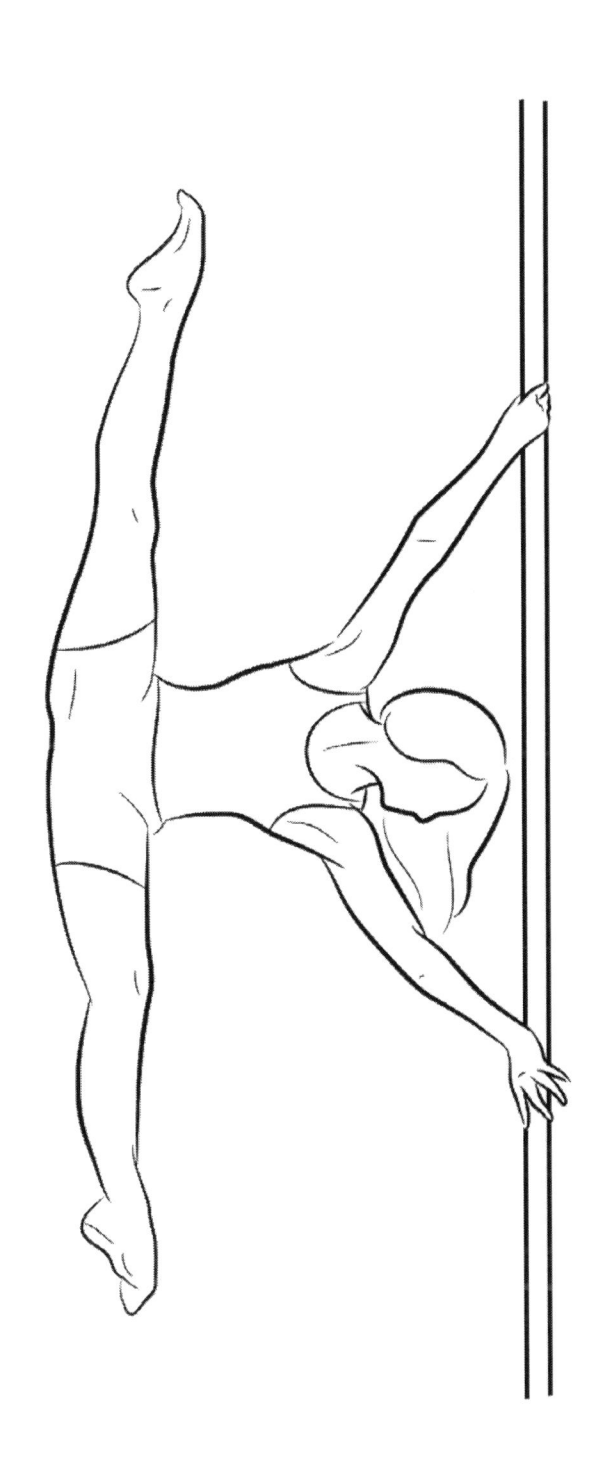

Extended Flexi Embrace

This is a great and fun flexible sort of pole move. You should make sure that you've built up your flexibility before you begin with this. To start, you want to climb up the pole, and from there, grip the pole with your right elbow. You should then, drop your legs so they're straight, allowing you to hang off the pole. From there, you should take your left hand, grip your right leg, and hold it, making a pretty shape. It's a great way to not only build a stretch, but it also looks very pretty as well.

With all of these movements, you can add them as transitions from the inverts and other movements. Often, posing works well too if you're wanting to work on a certain area, such as your elbows and other such areas that do require conditioning. With a few of these, they are of an easier level compared to the ones you might see. You should, however, work to try out all of these.

If you're struggling with grips, one of the best things to do is to get some pole cleaner, clean up the pole, get some pole tacky grip, put it on your arms and legs, along with our hands, and continue to use it as you work on the pole. It will help not only with keeping you there but also with making sure that you do maintain everything strength-wise.

Now that you know some poses, the best thing to do is learn to combine them. see how you can go from one to another, try to transition, adding in some of the floorwork, inverts, and other moves that you learned before. With each practice, with each step, you'll be one step closer to really mastering the pole, and with each and every sort of move, technique, and the like, you'll be able to build up your strength, which in turn will build up your confidence as well.

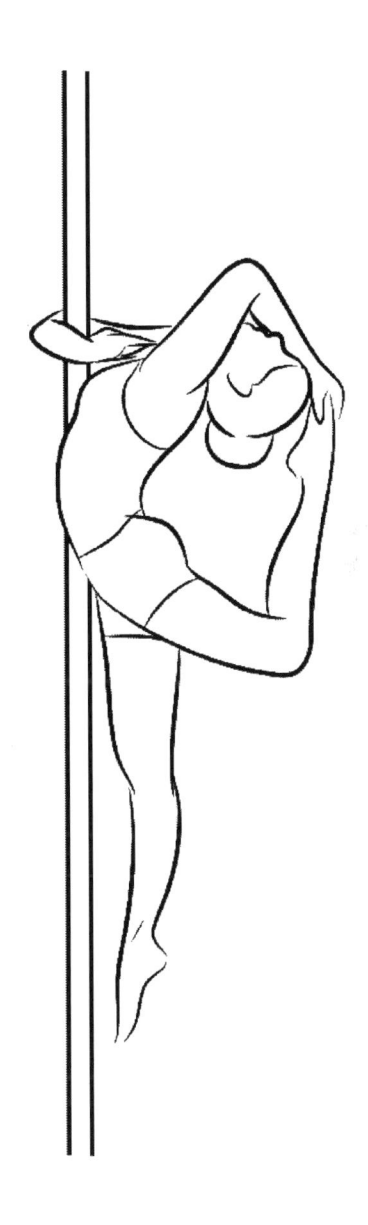

Extreme Doubles Actions to Master

Doubles moves are always a lot of fun, but at an extreme level, you need to ensure that both of you are in top shape. This chapter will go over some of the best doubles moves that you can master, and you'll see for yourself just what you can do to really master each of these.

One armed inverted one leg hang

This move is one that looks pretty but is also quite hard. The first one should get into an invert, taking their left leg and holding it there. From there, walk the back leg down, holding your hand out in order for the other person to come forward. Ideally, this one that is holding the hand should be able to maintain grip on the pole and hold the other person up.

For the one that is on the bottom, you have it kind of easier, you just need to be comfortable with putting your weight on the other person before you hold your leg to the pole. You should invert your body, and from there, bend one of your legs, and hold it against the pole if needed. Extend the other out, and then maintain the pose. Now, this can be quite hard for the bottom person as well, since holding your body up like that can be quite cumbersome, and since it's close to the ground, there is the risk of head injury. It's best to make sure that you can do this close to the ground before working with your partner on this move.

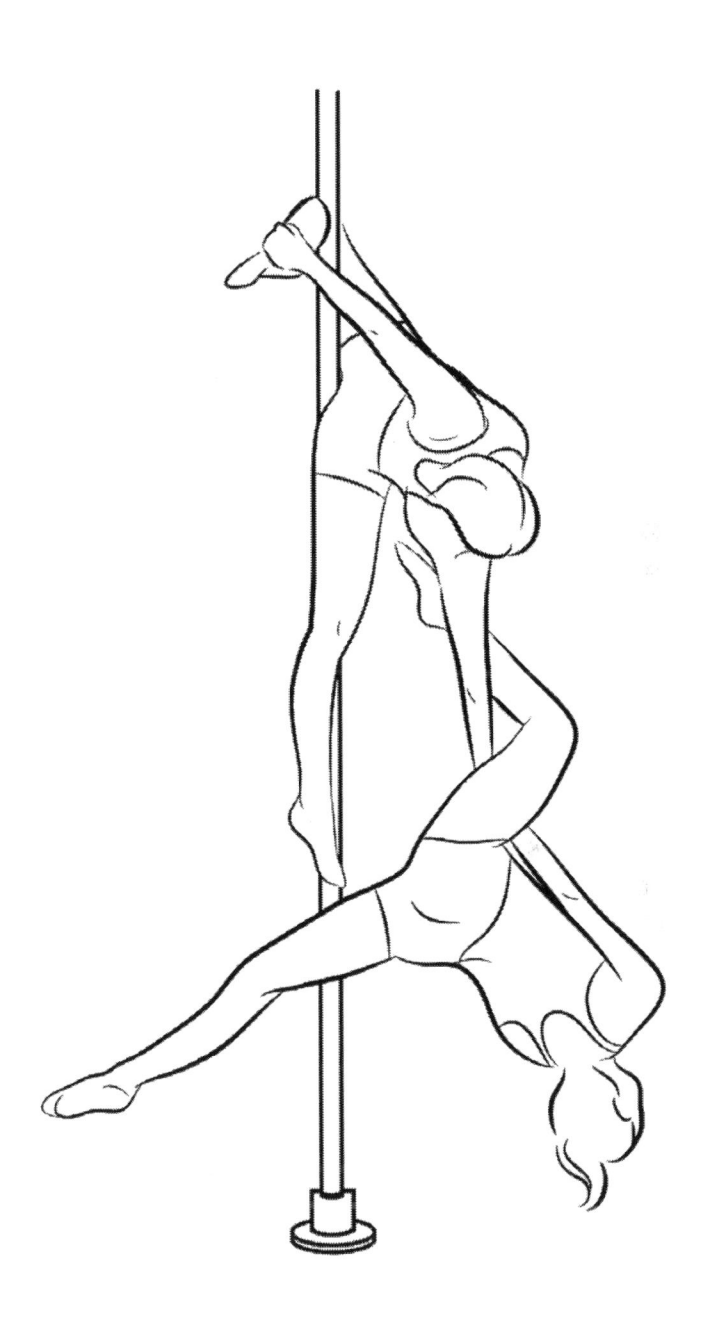

One arm inverted straddle

This is another fun move that you can try. To begin, it's the same as the first move, with one on top, and then, having the leg at the top of them bend down moving the bottom leg to a straightened position. You can then hold your legs to the pole, maintaining the grip. From there, the one on top should extend their hand, or if you want to be brave, both hands, using your legs to hold the pole. For the latter, make sure that you can do this with one hand on the pole since it is quite hard.

The one on the bottom has it much easier than on top, but again, it's the factor of being able to hold the position there. From there, they should get into an invert, straddling their legs this time and not having them on the pole. They should proceed to hold it there, maintaining the pressure and the grip as you continue on. This is a harder one, but it looks quite pretty.

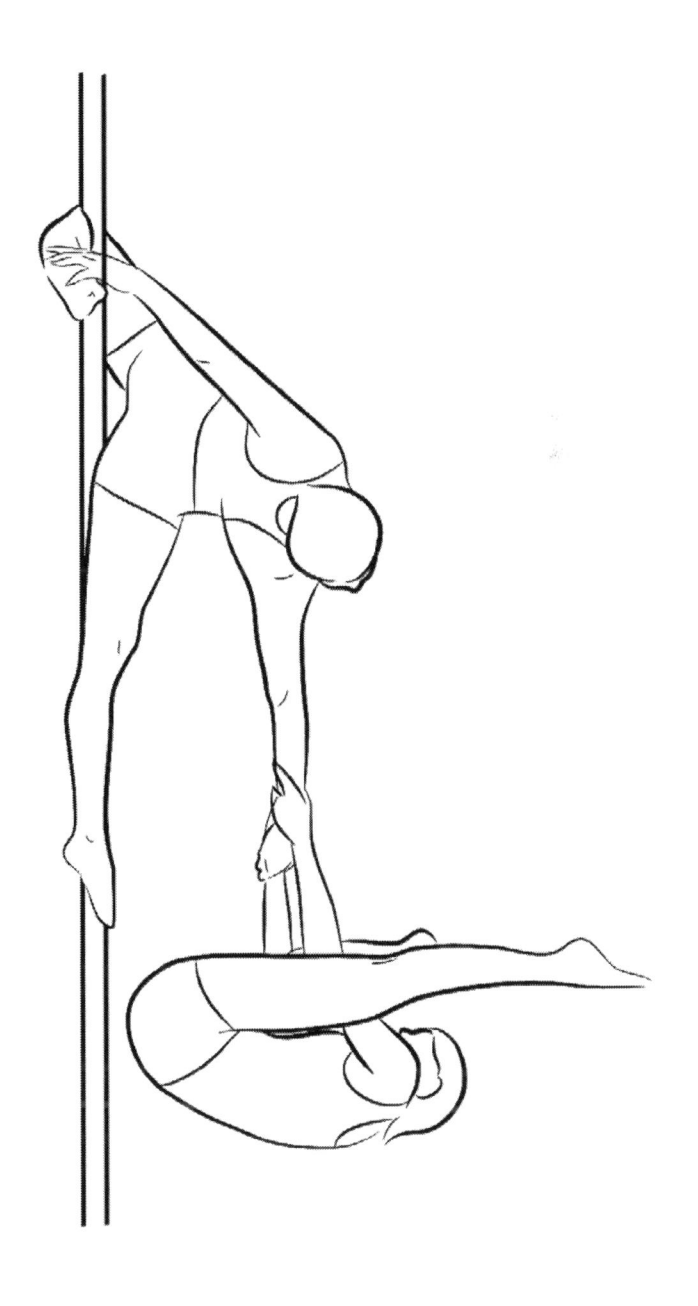

Circle

This circle is a fun move for two people, but it does require trust and some flexibility. To do this, you want to have one person go up, climbing the pole and from there, getting as high as possible, holding themselves onto the pole in a pole pose. From there, the one on the bottom should then proceed to go up, climbing the pole at the bottom, and from there, getting into either a u-bend or a superman, and then, climbing up to meet the other person.

For the top girl, you should start to fall back ripping the feet of the one below. The one on the bottom should do the same, extending their hands up and gripping the one on top. This is quite a complicated move, and often, it's definitely not something that many can do due to the constraints of space. However, once you learn it, it definitely is worth the effort.

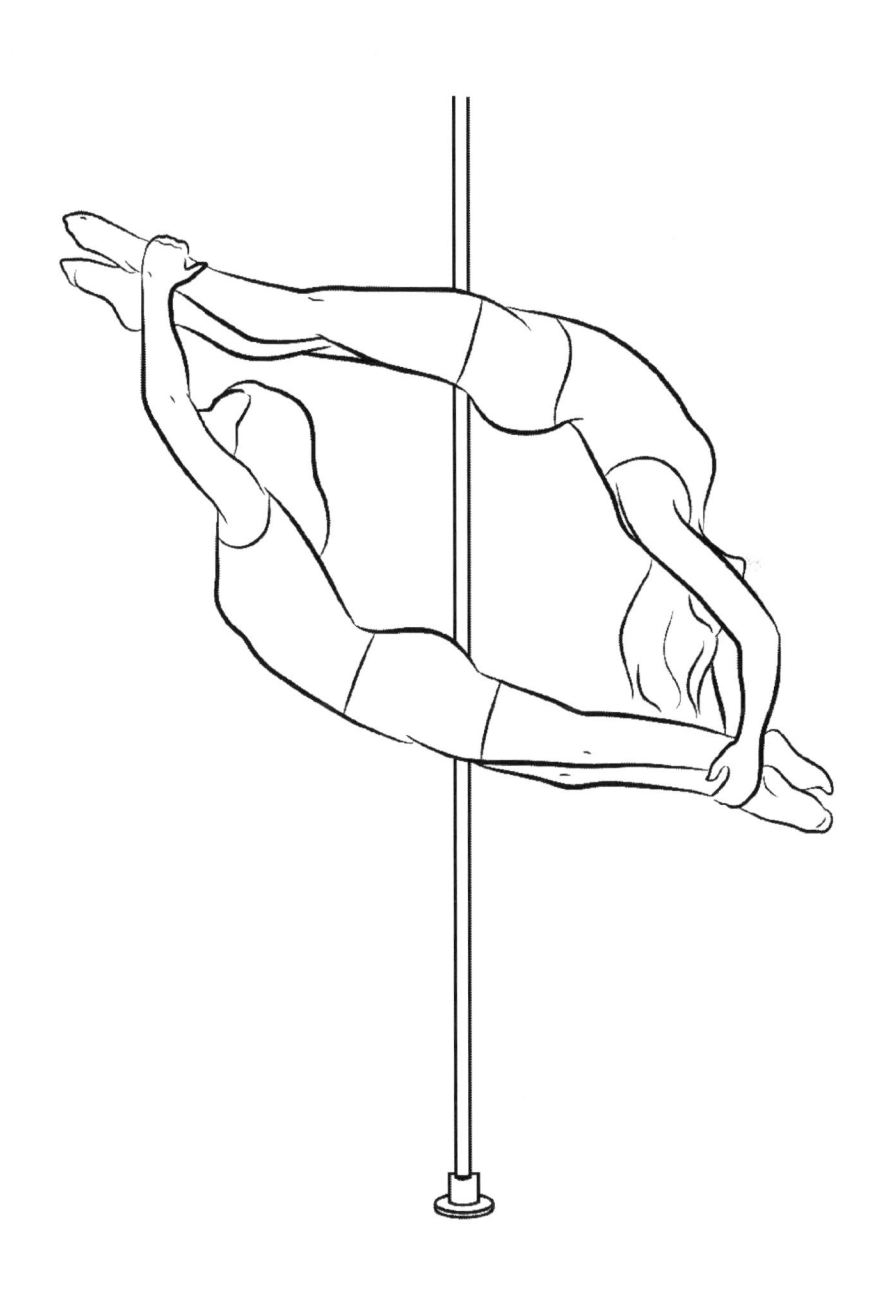

Two-Partnered Handspring

It's also called the Cuban Handspring. To do this one, you have to have one that isn't relatively flexible but is mostly strong, and the other who is able to do flexible actions, to begin, have one of you against the pole, legs a bit wider than shoulder width. Then, have one of your hands behind gripping the pole and the other on top, making a small hole with your elbow. For the one that is flexible, they should wrap their arm around the open hole, gripping the other's thigh to brace, and then lift their legs up, so that it's in a handspring formation. They can either have the legs spread or straight, and from there, simply hold the move. Once you're ready to come back down, you can.

This one is good if one of you is much more flexible and better at gymnastics-type moves than the other. If one of you is very strong, have them on the bottom, working to maintain the weight of the other person.

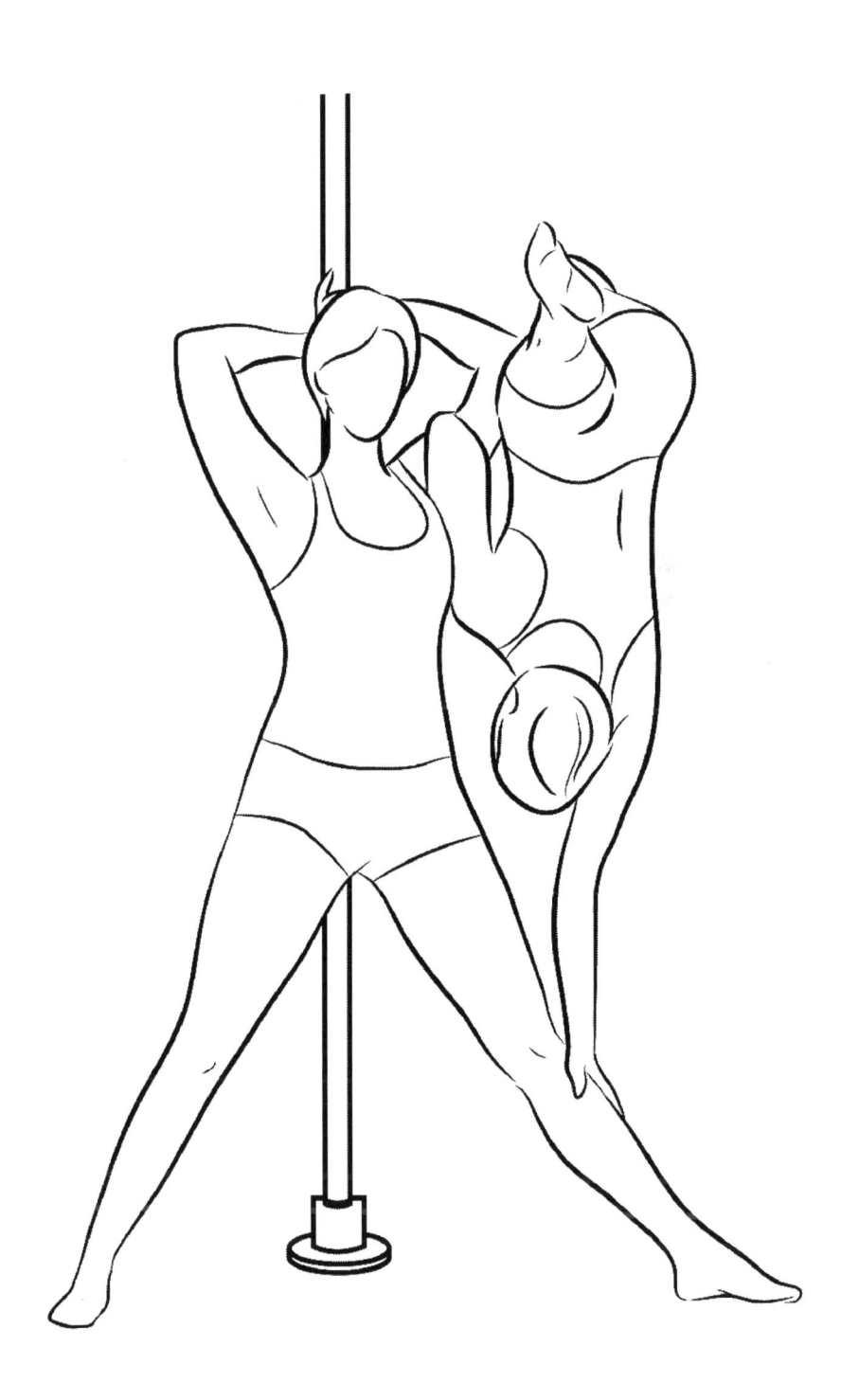

Death K

The Death Ka is quite a complicated, but very pretty, pole double move to try out. To being, you should have the one that will be on bottom stay near the bottom and hold the other body as they climb up on top. For the one on top, this is where your strength comes in, for you need to be able to get and maintain a shoulder mount as best as you can. The one on the bottom, once they're in that position, should quickly go from an invert, to a superman, and then have their body right up against the one that is on top. You will eventually be helping to keep the one on top up, and you should then spread your hands off into a death lay if you so desire. You don't have to, you can just grip the pole with one of your hands and then hold it there. From there, hold the move, maintain the position, and when ready, the one on the bottom should quickly get back into an invert and climb down, and the one on top can simply place their feet back down in order to get back to the ground.

These doubles moves are often very hard for you to learn, and they do require both trust and great strength. However, if you and a friend are interested in learning, then, by all means, try this. You may never know how far you might come if you do this, so try it out see for yourself just what you can achieve, and from there, you'll be able to add these to your repertoire of moves.

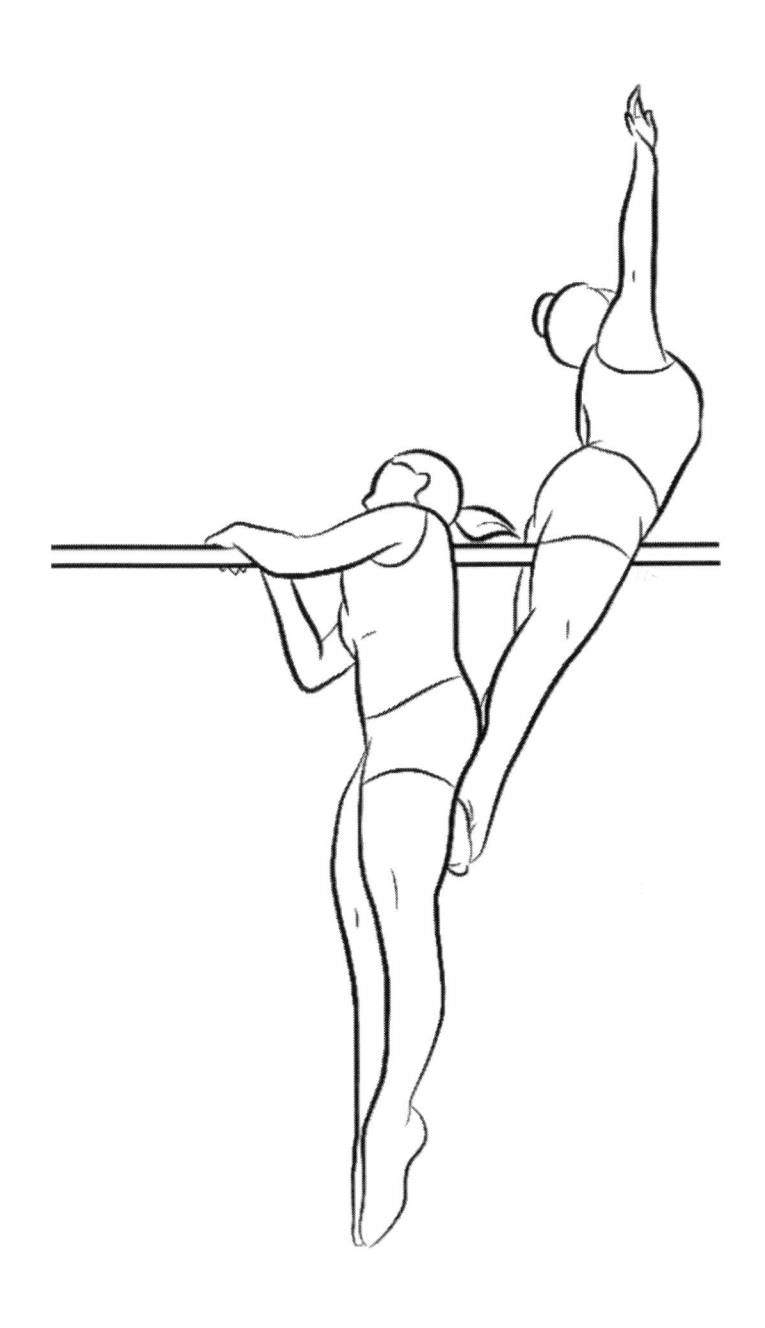

How to Build Flexibility

Often, the reason why you might not be hitting all of the moves you so desire is because you don't have your flexibility up to snuff. Flexibility is something that's integral to later pole moves, and often, it's something many don't work on, for they think they don't need it. but, if you're trying to hit the harder moves and you just can't do it, you can look to that as the culprit of the actions. You can up your training on this, especially in abdominal and arm strength, by becoming more flexible, and here are a few helpful tips to building this.

The first is you should listen to your body. If your body can't handle doing some sort of a stretch, or even a move, don't push yourself to do so. You might not be able to do everything right away, so don't push yourself too hard. That leads to problems.

Now, if you're going to stretch, you can do so after your workout. It's really for the best to do this afterward since you can really help with getting the distance further. You should make sure to work on this for a few minutes each and every single practice.

Now there are a few things that you can do. Touching your toes and gripping your hands and pulling them the opposite way is one thing. Ideally, stretching out your wrist by pushing it down palms facing the wall and just pushing can really help with this, but there are a few more to do.

There is the bridge, which is essentially you lie on your back on all fours. Lift your legs and feet up, holding it there.

You can also do it by getting into the splits position, or as far down as you can in the splits position. once you're able to do a jade split, you'll be able to reach back, gripping your back leg and holding it. You can bend it as well, and this will give you a great stretch in the legs.

Finally, there is the stretch where you lie on your stomach, bend your legs up in the air, and keeping your chest perpendicular to the ground. You can grab your legs from behind and bring them to your back as close as you can, holding them firmly and stretching. You'll want to make sure that you go all-out with this, because it gives your quads a killer workout as well, which is always a great thing.

You can also use the pole for a few flexibility and strength training options. I love to grab the pole with one of my hands, and my foot with another, bringing it back and holding it there. I love to feel the stretch, and it's definitely something I do enjoy. It's a great one for quads.

Finally, you can also try to use the pole for ab strength. If you're the type of person that wants to improve your abs. grasp the pole, hold it there, and then lower your legs as if you're going to do a leg drop. From there, hold it there firmly, grasping the pole and letting your legs stay about 6 inches off the ground. Try to hold this for at least a minute and then put them down. This is a great way to build that area up, and it does help a lot too.

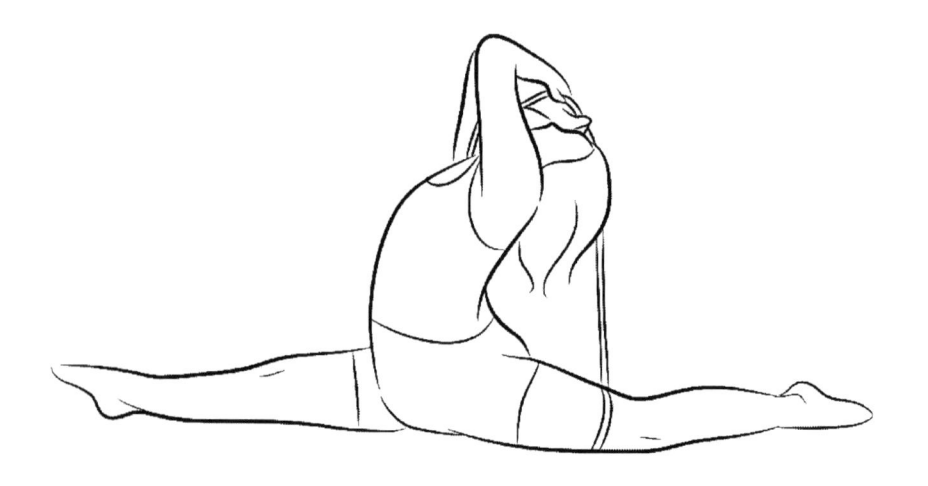

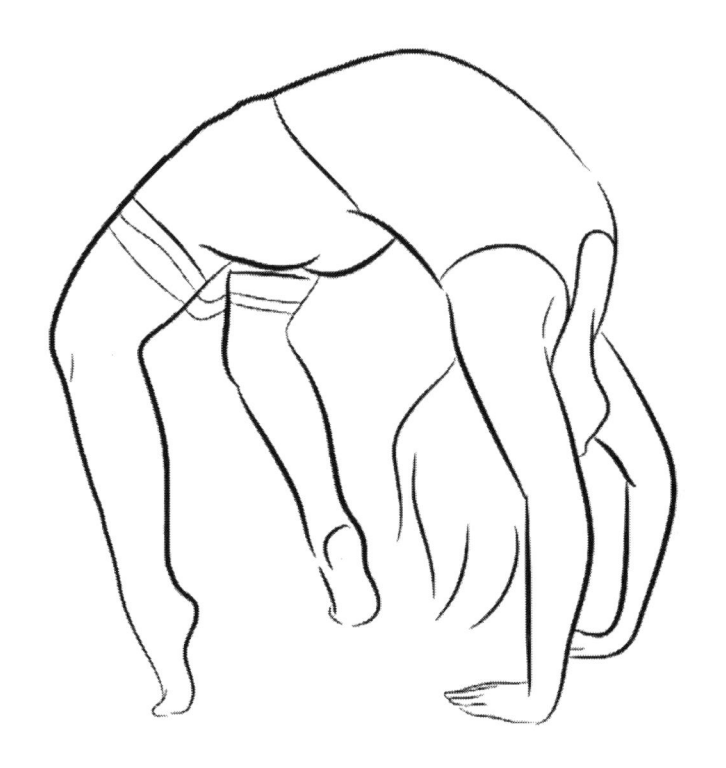

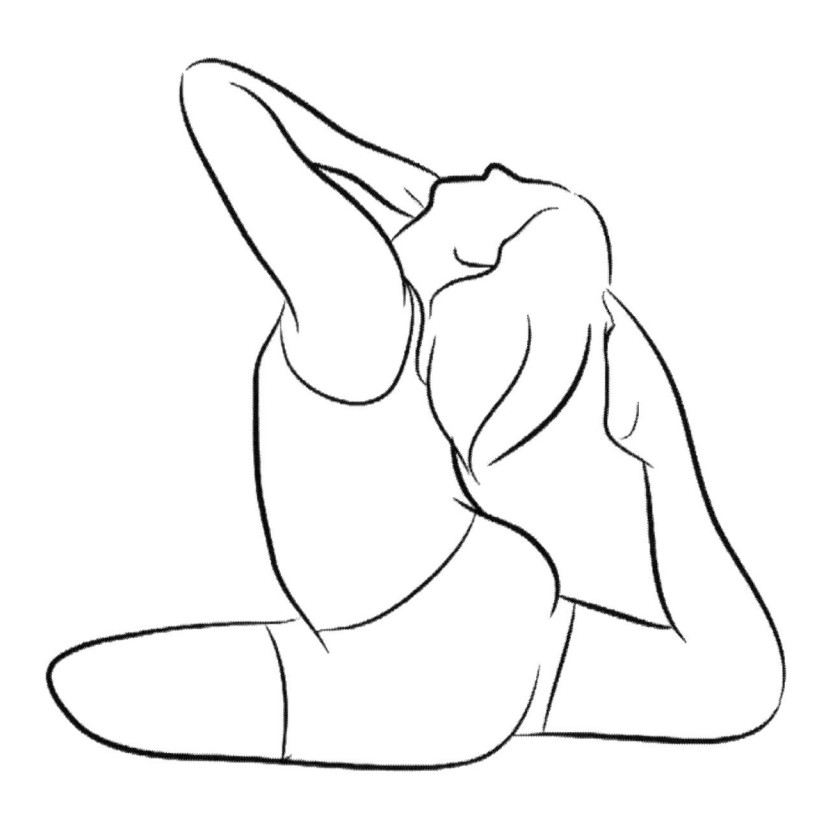

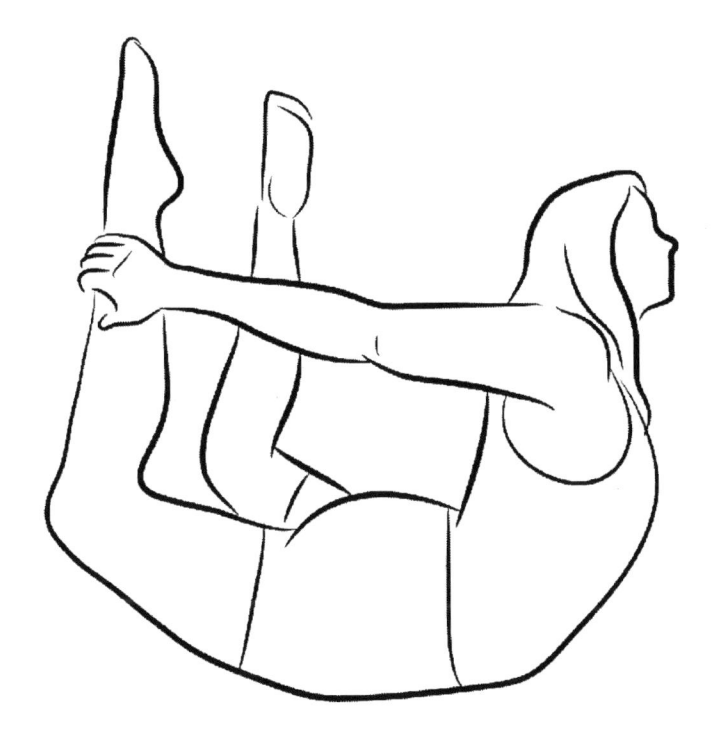

If you want to really stretch out your body, and you're feeling that typical stretches don't cut it, then try using a foam roller. You can use that to help with stretching your legs out. They're relatively cheap, and the results you get from this are simply magical. Stretching out your body is a great thing and almost essential to do in pole fitness. This chapter highlighted just why you do that, and some of the best ways to stretch for success

Tips to Help with Recording your Pole Moves

Now, recording your progress is essential to getting better as a pole dancer. You might hate this, but you can spot some of your flaws if you do this. Often, people don't realize they're doing basic things wrong with the pole and it's partially because they don't really realize that they have been doing this wrong the entire time. This chapter will go over some of the best ways to actually look at yourself, seeing what you need to do, and how to get good feedback on this as well.

Mirror, mirror

Mirrors are one of the best ways to actually see how you're doing on a pole. If you have the room in your studio or home, put it up. You can find these typically at a glass shop, a hardware or construction store, or a supply place that carries these. You should try to get one that actually isn't too pricey. These can run a lot, especially if they're fancy and framed, so make sure that you do take the time to find one that fits, mount it, and from there, use it to see how you're doing. This is a good way to correct anything that you see right away instead of waiting for a bit.

You don't have to use a mirror though. If you don't have the room, as in the case of if you're using your home as a pole studio, then you should try to figure out how to set up a video mount, and that's what we're going to discuss next.

Put it on Video

One of the biggest fears we all have is seeing yourself on video. It can be embarrassing, but with pole dancing, you want to make sure that you are doing the trick correctly, and not using a grip that could hurt yourself. You should try to record yourself a few times when you're trying to learn a new trick if you're doing it on your own without anyone to correct you. This is how all home pole training should be. Look at the trick, do the trick, and then compare it to the photo that you're using, such as the ones in this book. You'll be able to see from here what you need to do.

There are also some forums out there that you can use. There is one called the Studio Veena forum, which I've used before, in order to get feedback from both instructors and dancers alike.

This can be kind of embarrassing for you to do at first, and often, you might wonder if you're doing it okay. But you should definitely try to put it all together and see for yourself just where to focus. Often, we don't realize we're doing something wrong until somebody says so, and by then, it's often very hard to train ourselves out of that.

There are also some great recourses such as a training journal. A training journal is something that you can use in order to gauge your progress on your pole work. You can use a video recorder as well if you're really struggling with this. You can look at this every time you feel discouraged or frustrated, and you can see just how far you've come. There is a lot to which you can also gauge from this. If you feel like you're not learning a trick fast enough, look at this. You might see for yourself just how different everything is now. The trick that you're learning and are stuck on might actually be a trick that's ten times harder than the one you did a few months ago. It's a great way to really help you get the most out of your pole dancing, and you'll feel way better about your mistakes too.

Practice Makes Perfect

This is something that everyone should know, regardless if it's for pole dancing, or anything else. In order to do well with a sport, an activity, or whatever, you need to practice. Pole dancing is no exception, especially with everything that is happening. I know it's a bit discouraging, but remember, it takes courage to actually look at your mistakes and see what it is that you're doing wrong.

Often, when we first start, the idea of recording and seeing our mistakes can be utterly terrifying. But remember, if you don't work at it now, how are you ever going to get better with time.

The only way to improve in many cases is to suck it up and try on video. You might hate the way you look, the sound of your voice, and you might end up cringing every time you try to perform a trick. But think about it, if you don't do it now, will you ever get better? That's the thing, the only way to get better is to practice. You need to record yourself, need to learn from your mistakes, and become the best damn pole dancer you can be. Remember, you're in control of how you end up doing on your pole, and all of the tricks you learn, so it's best to learn fast and have fun with it.

This chapter went over the element of recording. Recording, in essence, is a bit of a scary action to undertake immediately, simply because the idea of recording your progress doesn't sound all that appealing. But remember, it's either learn now or re-learn everything later and often, getting it right the first time is a much better idea. So do that, learn your tricks, and most of all continue to have fun with this. The more you learn, the more you understand, and the more you try, the happier you'll be, and you'll see the results come to fruition in due time.

That's It!

This book taught you some pretty amazing new moves, from complex grip mounts to inverts, to even poses and doubles actions you can work on. You've seen through each of these pages and illustrations that while these moves are hard, they are totally doable.

For anyone really wanting to step up their pole dancing game, recording is where it is at too, and combining that, flexibility, and the moves listed here will make you into a fine pole dancer. if you're ready to take it seriously and try some of the expert moves, then your next step is to go for it.

Do practice. Work on it. Get friends to try it with you as well, and you'll soon see yourself evolve. You'll become the pole dancer you've wanted to be, a graceful artist that is ready to soar. So what are you waiting for? Get out there and start trying these.

One last thing! How awesome would it be if you shared your opinion about this book with a short review on Amazon? You read reviews yourself so why not give back a little to the community.

http://booksfor.review/expertpole

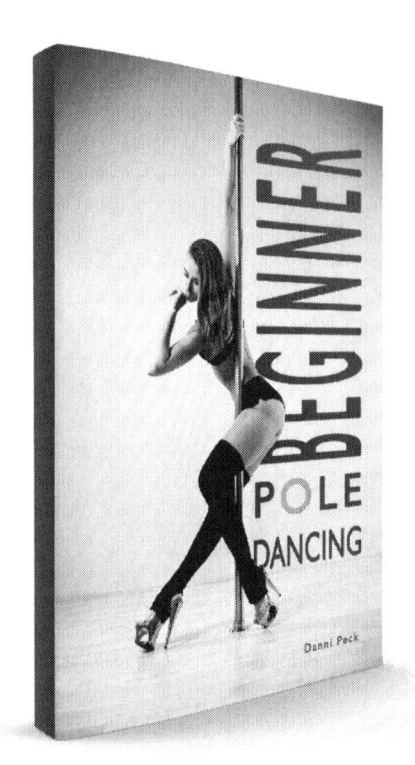

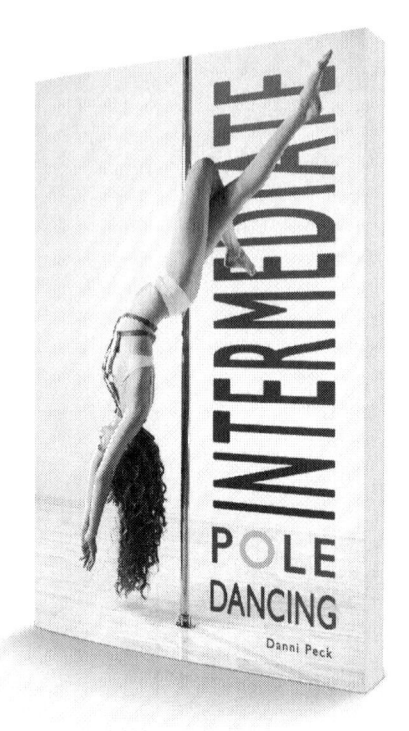

Available on Amazon

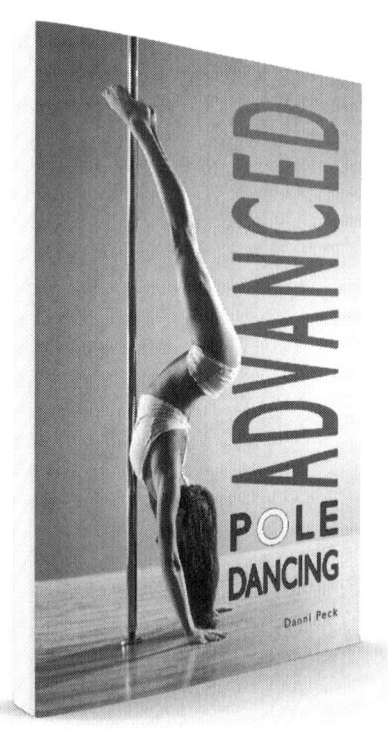

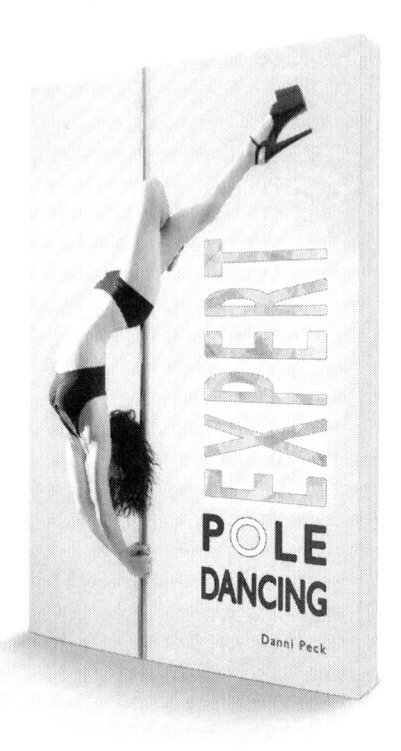

Page intentionally left blank.

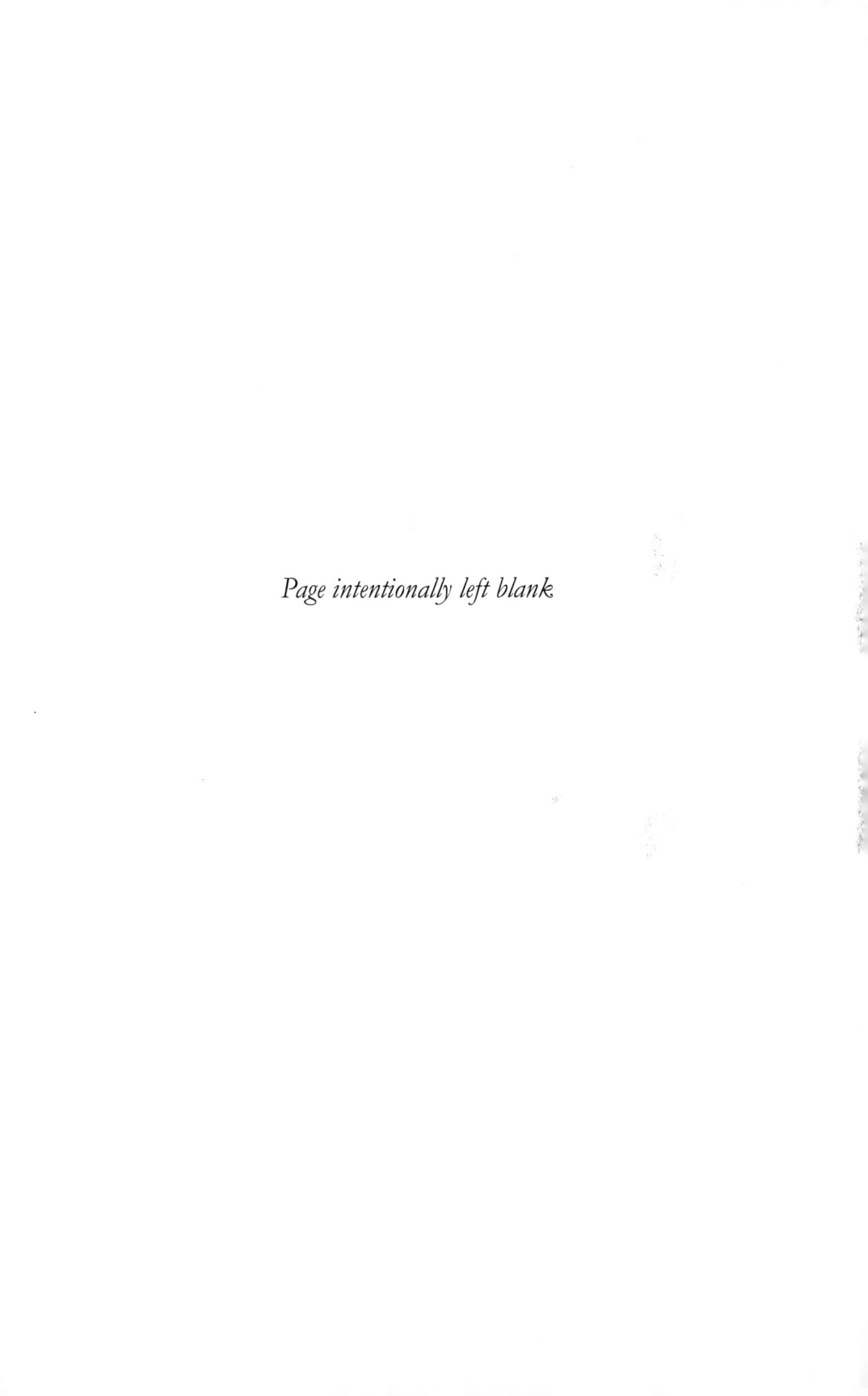

Printed in Great Britain
by Amazon